VOLUME XIII, NUMBER 2, APRIL 2014

D1245777

CLINICAL UPDATES IN WOMEN'S HEALTH CARE

Sexuality and Sexual Disorders

Rosemary Basson, MD, FRCP
Sexual Medicine Program
University of British Columbia
Vancouver, British Columbia

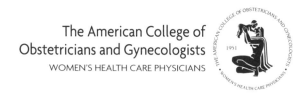

The American College of
Obstetricians and Gynecologists
WOMEN'S HEALTH CARE PHYSICIANS

Online access for subscribers—www.clinicalupdates.org

Clinical Updates in Women's Health Care is published quarterly by the American College of Obstetricians and Gynecologists (the College). This series represents the knowledge and experience of the authors and does not necessarily reflect the policy of the American College of Obstetricians and Gynecologists. The recommendations do not dictate an exclusive course of treatment or of practice. Variations taking into account the needs of the individual patient, resources, and limitations unique to the institution or type of practice may be appropriate.

ISSN: 1536-3619
ISBN: 978-1-934984-33-8

12345/87654   CU060

Contents

Sexuality and Sexual Disorders
Volume XIII, Number 2, April 2014
After reading *Sexuality and Sexual Disorders*, go to:
www.clinicalupdates.org

- Complete and submit the CME questions online—automatically add 5 CME credits to your College cognate transcript. CME credit is available for all titles posted online.

- View links to resources related to sexuality and sexual disorders.

  — American Association of Sexuality Educators, Counselors, and Therapists
    www.aasect.org

  — American Psychological Association: Aging and Human Sexuality Resource Guide
    www.apa.org/pi/aging/resources/guides/sexuality.aspx

  — International Society for the Study of Women's Sexual Health
    www.isswsh.org

  — The Kinsey Institute
    www.indiana.edu/~kinsey

  — National Vulvodynia Association
    www.nva.org

  — North American Menopause Society
    www.menopause.org

  — Sexuality Information and Education Council of the United States
    www.siecus.org

  — Society for Sex Therapy and Research
    www.sstarnet.org

- Order College patient education material.

- See full text of past issues and any relevant changes or updates.

Continuing Medical Education

Objectives

This monograph is designed to enable obstetrician–gynecologists to do the following:

- Integrate the biologic and psychologic factors that underlie women's sexual response and sexual dysfunction
- Screen patients for sexual disorders
- Identify risk factors for sexual dysfunction, including gynecologic conditions and therapeutic interventions
- Evaluate patients who have sexual disorders and initiate or indicate management
- Explain current uncertainty regarding testosterone supplementation or investigational pharmacologic therapy for sexual dysfunction
- Identify when referral to a mental health provider is needed
- Refer patients to patient education resources

ACCME Accreditation

The American College of Obstetricians and Gynecologists is accredited by the Accreditation Council for Continuing Medical Education (ACCME) to provide continuing medical education for physicians.

AMA PRA Category 1 Credit(s)™

The American College of Obstetricians and Gynecologists designates this enduring activity for a maximum of *5 AMA PRA Category 1 Credit(s)™*. Physicians should only claim credit commensurate with the extent of their participation in the activity.

College Cognate Credit(s)

The American College of Obstetricians and Gynecologists designates this enduring activity for a maximum of 5 Category 1 College Cognate Credit(s). The College has a reciprocity agreement with the AMA that allows **AMA PRA Category 1 Credit(s)™** to be equivalent to College Cognate Credits.

Credit for *Clinical Updates in Women's Health Care: Sexuality and Sexual Disorders*, Volume XIII, Number 2, April 2014, is initially available through December 2017. During that year, the unit will be re-evaluated. If the content remains current, credit is extended for an additional 3 years.

Disclosure Statement

Current guidelines state that continuing medical education (CME) providers must ensure that CME activities are free from the control of any commercial interest. All authors, editorial board members, and reviewers declare that neither they nor any business associate nor any member of their immediate families has material interest, financial interest, or other relationships with any company manufacturing commercial products relative to the topics included in this publication or with any provider of commercial services discussed in this publication except for Raul Artal, MD, who has been involved with clinical trials with Nascent, Solvay, Xenodyne, Symbollon Pharmaceuticals, and Columbia Laboratories and Julia Schlam Edelman, MD, who has financial interests in Alnylam Pharmaceuticals and Intelligent Bio-Systems. Any conflicts have been resolved through group and outside review of all content.

See page v for submission of CME credits.

Foreword

In 2003, we published a monograph on the topic of sexuality and sexual disorders written by Dr. Rosemary Basson, a recognized world authority on the subject. Since that publication, new information, understanding, and therapeutic approaches have occurred. Dr. Basson has now written an update that outlines changes in the classification of sexual disorders and a holistic approach to their management. New research has been conducted in the time since the last publication, and the author discusses the results of this research and how they have modified our understanding of sexual disorders. This monograph is a useful tool for all physicians who provide health care to women because it will help them better understand and manage these important conditions, which affect the patient's quality of life.

Morton A. Stenchever, MD
Editor Emeritus

ABSTRACT: This monograph describes the physiology of women's sexual response, particularly the interplay of psychologic and biologic factors: the mind modulates physiology; disease affects the psyche. The current understanding of women's sexual response cycles, including the concepts of sexual motivation and sexual arousability, are presented to clarify the etiology and evolution of common types of sexual dysfunction and to provide management guidelines. Changes in sexuality through the life cycle are addressed. Principles and methods to assess sexual concerns and diagnose sexual problems, including disorders of sexual interest, arousal, and orgasm, are outlined, as are risk factors for sexual dysfunction. This update also includes discussions of the management of pain from estrogen deficiency and provoked vestibulodynia and nonconsummation of relationship from fear of vaginal penetration. The uncertainty regarding androgen supplementation also is discussed.

Sexuality is basic to the human condition, and women rate sexuality as important to their quality of life (1). Evidence exists that a healthy sexual life encourages taking care of general health concerns and adopting a healthy lifestyle (2). Untreated sexual dysfunction associated with past sexual, physical, and emotional abuse can perpetuate the cycle of poor self-esteem, promiscuity, depression, substance abuse, a variety of physical problems that defy a clear diagnosis, and an inability to trust other individuals, especially those of the same sex as the perpetrators. Studies suggest that physicians are mostly unaware of the nature and severity of the sexual concerns of their patients—approximately 70–80% of postmenopausal women with dyspareunia had not discussed this condition with their physicians (3, 4).

The obstetrician–gynecologist's role in assessing patients' sexual function and dysfunction, initiating treatment, and making appropriate referrals is crucial because women view their sexuality as being frequently affected by reproductive events. Moreover, gynecologic disease processes and therapeutic interventions can potentially harm sexual response. Although sexual function is an important contributor to sexual satisfaction, other factors also are involved (eg, relationship [5, 6], intrapersonal variables [especially mood], self-image, and stress [7, 8]). Dysfunction does not necessarily lead to dissatisfaction (9).

Management of sexual problems by obstetrician–gynecologists may include the following components:

- Providing basic detailed information regarding the sexual response cycle and underlying physiology

- Assessing factors that contribute to sexual interest/arousal disorder to direct therapy or to advise sexual and nonsexual behavioral changes for the couple

- Assessing and managing chronic dyspareunia or apareunia

- Prescribing medication or hormone therapy (HT)

- Advising caution regarding the lack of safety and benefit data for some products that claim to improve sexual dysfunction

Epidemiology

Epidemiologic studies report high prevalence of women with sexual dysfunction in the United States (30–40% of women), but these figures are reduced to some 10% if dysfunction is accompanied by distress (10). Sexual distress is linked to depression and relationship factors (11). Survey questionnaires are based on outdated definitions of sexual disorders that are more reflective of male sexuality (eg, absence of sexual fantasies and desire before sexual engagement as implying disorder) and have proved problematic (12). For example, in one study of 400 women who completed questionnaires in family practice offices, similar numbers of women (approximately 20% for each group) received the diagnosis of sexual dysfunction but reported no problems, did not receive the diagnosis but reported problems, and received diagnosis and agreed they perceived a problem (13).

Of women who live in the United States, the prevalence of reported sexual dysfunction is higher in those of Japanese and Chinese backgrounds and lower in African American women (14). Globally, the highest prevalence of sexual dysfunction occurs in women who live in East Asia, Southeast Asia, and the Middle East compared with those who live in Europe and North America (15). Prevalence figures from nationally representative surveys of U.S. women suggest a prevalence of hypoactive sexual desire disorder of 8.3% and 9.4% with minimal variation across age groups other than a decrease in women older than 60 years (5.8%) (16). Prevalence of hypoactive sexual desire disorder reaches 12.5% in surgically menopausal women generally and 19.8% in those younger than 45 years (16). Most surveys have focused on the lubrication component of arousal dysfunction as opposed to problems with subjective excitement or arousal; a large survey of women older than 40 years showed that approximately 17% of women reported moderately or highly problematic arousal (17). Strict use of the distress criteria suggests a prevalence of orgasmic disorder of 3.3%; 9.3% of 987 women assessed did not experience orgasm (18). In nonclinical samples, 18–20% of premenopausal women have chronic dyspareunia (19, 20), and studies of dyspareunia in postmenopausal women show prevalence rates of 20–44% (14, 21–23). One study noted that only one third of the 50% of women with moderate to severe symptoms sought medical care (24); another study noted that a belief that this was a normal part of aging was the most common reason for not seeking care (23). Research suggests lesbian and bisexual women have similar but fewer types of sexual dysfunction than heterosexual women (25). Low desire or desire discrepancy (ie, both partners' desire considered to be within normal range but one consistently higher), are the most common concerns. Concerns about insufficient lubrication and dyspareunia have been considered to be less common in lesbian and bisexual women than in heterosexual women. However, results of an online survey suggest otherwise—32 out of 32 lesbians reported pain with vulval and vaginal stimulation (26). Orgasmic difficulty is less frequent in these women than in other populations. Ease of orgasm is related to time spent on sex, and this fact is true for both lesbian and heterosexual women (25). Another large

online survey of women who have had sex with women, suggests that risk factors for sexual dysfunction may be different
than those operating in the population of women who have not
had sex with women; eg, partner factors affected sexual function
but not sexual interest or desire (27). Transgender women mostly
are pleased with the sexual outcome of sex reassignment surgery,
but orgasmic dysfunction and difficulties with neovaginal penile
intercourse may be reported to the gynecologist (28).

Risk Factors

Sexual disorders may be identified during visits for routine gynecologic care. In addition, women with certain conditions have a
high prevalence of specific sexual disorders (Box 1).

Effects of Life Cycle and Reproductive Events

Sexual function may be affected by many of the biologic and psychologic aspects of reproduction and the life cycle. These events
are listed in Box 2. All of these factors can interfere with sexual
function, but how commonly they do so is unknown. The mechanisms governing the interplay between psychologic responses to
reproductive events and the biologic changes themselves are not
well understood. However, women's past sexual experiences,
self-image, support from and attraction to their sexual partners,
knowledge of sexuality, and sense of control are all typically
important factors.

PREGNANCY

Given the multiple factors that affect a woman's sexuality, including her relationship, self-image, energy level, mood, cultural background, and hormonal status, changes in sexual function during
pregnancy and the postpartum period are numerous. A meta-
analysis showed that 90% of women were sexually active during
pregnancy, but this number decreased to approximately one third
by the ninth month (29). By the third trimester "dysfunction"
was common enough that it really could be considered normative (approximately 90% of women reported diminished clitoral
sensation, loss of desire, or difficulties with orgasm in a study
of 589 pregnant women) (30). Although 14.7% and 14.1% of

Box 1. Risk Factors

☑ Depression, with or without the use of anti-depressants*

☑ Anxiety disorder*

☑ Breast cancer that required chemotherapy

☑ Nonnerve-sparing radical hysterectomy or cystectomy

☑ Psychologic sequelae of gynecologic cancer and breast cancer

☑ Premature ovarian failure

☑ Neurologic disease

☑ Hypertension

☑ Diabetes

☑ Sexual abuse*

☑ Relationship discord*

☑ Partner sexual dysfunction

☑ Stress—emotional or environmental*

☑ Personality traits of perfectionism and self-dislike

☑ Negative sexual attitudes

*Robust evidence of risk exists.

women excluded intercourse in the first and second trimesters, respectively, for a variety of reasons, such as fear of precipitating labor, fear of harming the fetus, or cultural reasons, 41% excluded sexual intercourse from any sexual activity by the third trimester (30) (see Box 3).

Postpartum Period

Dyspareunia. High-quality evidence is lacking to support that either vaginal or abdominal birth results in better postpartum

---

Box 2. Effects of Life Cycle and Reproductive Events on Sexual Function

- Healthy pregnancy
- Complicated pregnancy during which sexual intercourse and orgasm are precluded
- Postpartum period
- Recurrent pregnancy loss
- Therapeutic abortion
- Infertility
- Perimenopause
- Natural menopause
- Premature menopause (idiopathic and iatrogenic)

---

sexual function. Studies have shown that perineal trauma and operative vaginal delivery are associated with postpartum dyspareunia and other types of sexual dysfunction. For example, one study found that women with a second-degree laceration had an 80% increase of dyspareunia at 3 months postpartum compared with women who gave birth with an intact perineum. Women with third- or fourth-degree lacerations had a 270% increased likelihood of dyspareunia (31). Similarly, the relative risk of not resuming sexual intercourse by 6 months is higher in women who had lacerations in the vagina, perineum, sphincter ani, or rectum than in women who gave birth with an intact perineum (32).

It is uncertain if operative vaginal deliveries and dyspareunia and other types of sexual dysfunction are associated with the lacerations at the time of delivery, an episiotomy, or the operative delivery itself. One study showed an increased odds ratio of 2.5 for dyspareunia at 6 months postpartum in women who underwent operative delivery compared with those who underwent nonoperative vaginal delivery, after controlling for the depth of perineal laceration, length of the second stage of labor, interval between deliveries, and any prior history of dyspareunia (31).

Box 3. Risks of Sexual Activity in Pregnancy

- Preterm Labor
  Risk factors include previous preterm labor, multiple gestation, cervical incompetence (minimal data to support these risk factors), and lower genital tract infection*

- Antepartum Hemorrhage in Placenta Previa
  Theoretical risk of catastrophic antepartum hemorrhage[†] from intercourse or orgasm has been reported. Studies of the safety of transvaginal ultrasound probes in the setting of placenta previa are reassuring.[‡]

- Pelvic Inflammatory Disease
  Risk factor is unprotected sex—sexually transmitted disease that leads to pelvic inflammatory disease from ascending infection is possible in the first trimester. Theoretical protection after the twelfth week of gestation includes mucus plug and obliteration of the uterine cavity by fusion of the decidua capsularis and parietalis.

- Venous Air Embolism
  Venous air embolism is rare, but risk factors include oral–genital sex with air insufflation and penile–vaginal intercourse in the rear entry position where the level of the uterus is above the level of the heart.[¶]

*Read JS, Klebanoff MA. Sexual intercourse during pregnancy and preterm delivery: effects of vaginal microorganisms. The Vaginal Infections and Prematurity Study Group. Am J Obstet Gynecol 1993;168:514–9.

[†]Jones C, Chan C, Farine D. Sex in pregnancy. CMAJ 2011;183:815–8.

[‡]Timor-Tritsch IE, Yunis RA. Confirming the safety of transvaginal sonography in patients suspected of placenta previa. Obstet Gynecol 1993;81:742–4.

[¶]Lyness JR, Bentley AJ. Air embolism during sexual intercourse in the puerperium. Am J Forensic Med Pathol 2010;31:247–9.

Judicious use of operative vaginal delivery, possibly limiting episiotomy, and antenatal perineal massage may result in fewer severe perineal lacerations. However, the effects of these interventions on sexual function are unclear. Possibly the details of the suturing are important; for instance, not suturing through perineal skin during a repair has been shown to decrease postpartum perineal pain (33). Pelvic floor exercises during pregnancy and the postpartum period have been associated with less urinary and anal incontinence at 12 months—both of these factors potentially negatively influence sexual function (34). It has been reported that women who began pelvic floor muscle strengthening exercises in their fourth postpartum month had better sexual function in the seventh postpartum month compared with women in a control group (34).

Sexual Dysfunction Associated With Postpartum Depression. Depression has been found to be associated with loss of sexual interest at 8–12 weeks postpartum and at 6 months postpartum (35). In women with a history of depression, a significant decrease in sexual interest and satisfaction was documented even after the depression had resolved (29). When sexual dysfunction appears to be attributable to treatment with selective serotonin reuptake inhibitors (SSRIs), provided that the woman is not breastfeeding, the medication might be changed to bupropion or mirtazapine. The safety profile of bupropion use during breastfeeding is uncertain—the level of exposure appears to be minimal, and few data are available on the safety of mirtazapine.

Breastfeeding and Sexual Function. Increased prolactin levels lead to decreased ovarian production of estrogen. Some studies have found breastfeeding to be associated with an increased odds ratio (4.4) of dyspareunia at 6 months postpartum (31). Release of oxytocin (typically during breastfeeding) may result in sexual arousal, which might be uncomfortable for some women. It is helpful for clinicians to discuss this ahead of time and explain that it is normal. Similarly, oxytocin release with the uterine contractions of orgasms may result in milk ejection even during pregnancy and most typically during the postpartum period. Especially early in the postpartum period, frequent breastfeeding and the neediness of the infant compounded by fatigue often lessen the woman's desire for sexual or even nonsexual affectionate physical contact. Again, the normality of these experiences can be discussed.

Not being sexually active at 12 weeks of pregnancy is predictive of dissatisfaction with the sexual relationship 1 year postpartum. This underlies the importance of discussing sexual problems early in pregnancy (Box 4) (36).

MENOPAUSE

Some cross-sectional studies have shown that menopause can negatively affect sexual functioning (independent of aging), but other studies give conflicting results (37–40). In an 8-year longitudinal study of Australian women, data from the four groups of

---

Box 4. Addressing Sexuality During Pregnancy and the Postpartum Period

- Provide information of normative changes of pregnancy and the postpartum period
- Clarify any risks of sexual activity
- Clarify that nonpenetrative sex is part of normal sexual activity and very common in later stages of pregnancy and the postpartum period if dyspareunia is present
- Discuss the option of perineal massage to minimize perineal trauma and postpartum pain
- Before delivery, initiate discussion of birth control
- Address pelvic floor muscle training during pregnancy and the postpartum period
- Address mood issues throughout pregnancy and the postpartum period
- Explain that low desire is a normal occurrence in the postpartum period
- Encourage the use of vaginal lubricants or topical vaginal estrogen in the postpartum period

women were analyzed: 1) premenopausal, 2) postmenopausal, 3) early perimenopausal, and 4) late perimenopausal women for the duration of the study (37). The total score for sexual function, which included responsiveness, feelings for their partners, frequency of sex, desire, and absence of dyspareunia and sexual problems in their partners, decreased with the transition into menopause. Most changes in sexual function occurred between early perimenopause and late perimenopause, with further smaller overall reductions that occurred in the transitional period from late perimenopause to postmenopause. Dyspareunia and sexual dysfunction in partners increased markedly in the period from late perimenopause to postmenopause. Sexual responsiveness decreased with aging and menopause. With the use of different statistical techniques, estrogen status was found to be related to dyspareunia and to the number of menopausal symptoms, including insomnia and hot flushes. These symptoms affected well-being that, in turn, affected sexual desire and responsiveness. Women's feelings for their partners exerted a powerful effect on sexual desire. Daily hassles and interpersonal problems also affected well-being and, therefore, indirectly affected sexual responsiveness and desire.

A cross-sectional study of women who did not receive HT has shown the lowest levels of desire to be reported by perimenopausal women (38). Postmenopausal women reported decreased arousal compared with their status in the early fourth decade of their lives, but their menopausal status was unrelated to other aspects of sexual functioning in either unadjusted or multiple regression analysis (38). Low serum estradiol levels were related only to pain. Factors, such as physical health, new partners, mental health, and smoking, had a greater effect on women's sexual functioning than their menopausal status. Sexual satisfaction increased if their partners had physical limitations that caused them to reduce the frequency of sex.

A recent longitudinal study of Seattle women identified a small decrease in desire across the menopausal transition, and this was related to stress, vasomotor symptoms, sleep disturbance, mood, and fatigue but not to vaginal dryness (39). Exercise, perceived health status, alcohol consumption, and not having a long-term partner were linked to increased desire.

Another cross-sectional study has identified the role of intimacy in mediating negative effects of menopause on sexual desire and function. The postmenopausal state was associated with decreased desire but mostly among women who reported low intimacy with their sexual partners (40).

Women with premature menopause had decreased sexual arousal and increased genital pain compared with women in the control group in one study (41). Of note, they also had increased rates of anxiety, depression, and psychologic distress.

Approximately 16–20% of women younger than 49 years reported low desire subsequent to recommended surgical menopause (some procedures would likely have been for malignancy and some may have imposed unwanted infertility) (42, 43). However, women with elective bilateral oophorectomy who required hysterectomy for benign disease in midlife were not found to develop sexual dysfunction in the next 3 years (44, 45).

Sexual Response

In evaluating sexual problems, an understanding of female sexual response is needed. Sexual function and dysfunction are perhaps the supreme examples of a mandatory blending of mind and body—this interaction is crucial to the understanding of assessment and management of sexual problems. The outdated dualistic approach that dysfunction is psychologic, biologic, or psychologic plus biologic limits the understanding of female sexuality; matters of the mind affect physiology, and disease affects the psyche.

Sexual Response Cycle

Sexual desire (as in "drive" or "urge") is just one of many reasons women (and men) initiate or agree to have sexual intercourse (46). Middle-aged women have more motives than younger women, but their main focus remains love, commitment, and pleasure, motives shown to relate positively to women's sexual satisfaction (47). Women's desire, potentially absent at the outset of sexual activity, can be triggered subsequently during the sexual encounter. Data from 125 women aged 20–70 years showed that whether premenopausal or postmenopausal and whether reporting sexual dysfunction or not, all women identified triggers of sexual desire (48). These triggers were in the domains of emotional bonding, erotica, romance, and physical proximity. An absence of any initial desire was shown in the baseline Study of Women Across the Nation, where most of 3,262 multi-ethnic middle-aged women in North America indicated that although they were moderately or extremely satisfied with their physical sexual pleasure, they never or infrequently sensed desire (14). The highest figures were for Chinese and Japanese women (61.4% and 67.8%).

Of 3,687 women who completed a web-based survey, 1,865 women were deemed sexually functional with easy sexual arousal. Within this "functional" group, close to one third of women rarely or never began a sexual experience with a sense of sexual desire; it reliably was accessed once they were aroused (49). Only 15% of women in the "functional" group limited sexual activity to times they felt desire at the outset. Consistent anticipatory sexual desire is more typical of new relationships than old relationships, and as such, it may be a major reason for sexual engagement (49). Thus, current conceptualization of female (and male) sexual response allows for the possibility that a willingness to become aroused occurs first and is followed by sensing desire (Fig. 1). Empirical support for the concept that arousal may precede desire and the two then coexist is now strong and includes data from older and younger women (49–52). The proposed definition of sexual disorder in the American Psychiatric Association's *Diagnostic and Statistical Manual of Mental Disorders*, Fifth Edition (*DSM-5*), merges women's sexual interest (motivation) and arousal and focuses away from initial or anticipatory desire (53). Validated questionnaires used to assess sexual function are based on models of sexual response in which desire is assumed necessary at the outset of engagement. This is now acknowledged as a serious limitation to research (12).

Sexual Arousal

In the past, women's sexual arousal often was equated with vaginal lubrication. This unconscious reflex organized by the autonomic nervous system in response to mental or physical stimuli that are recognized as sexual is but one aspect of sexual arousal.

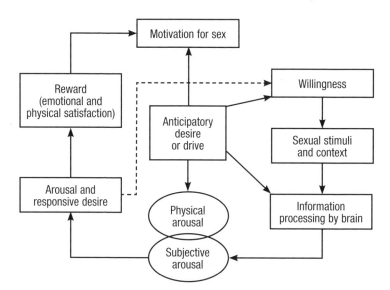

Fig. 1. Circular sexual response cycle shows overlapping phases of variable order. Reasons or motivations for sex are numerous, and sexual desire or drive may or may not be present at the outset but reached after the brain has processed sexual signals as sexual arousal, which conflates with sexual desire. The latter creates an urge for increased arousal, allowing acceptance of increasingly intense sexual stimulation.

Overall, subjective sexual arousal is a product of the following components:

- Mental sexual excitement—proportional to how exciting the woman finds the sexual stimulus and context
- Vulvar congestion—direct awareness (tingling and throbbing) is highly variable
- Pleasure from stimulating the engorging vulva
- Vaginal congestion—the woman's direct awareness is highly variable
- Pleasure from stimulating congested anterior vaginal wall and surrounding tissue
- Increased and modified lubrication—wetness per se usually is not directly arousing to the woman
- Vaginal nonvascular smooth muscle relaxation—usually, women are minimally aware of this

- Pleasure from stimulating nongenital areas of the body

- Other somatic changes—increased blood pressure, heart rate, muscle tone, respiratory rate, and temperature

The extent to which each component of sexual arousal contributes to the subjective experience currently is being studied. In men, genital vasocongestion can be considered a secondary confirmatory stimulus. Typically, men are accurately aware of that congestion and find it sexually exciting. However, in women, congestion may not register at all or only minimally, may not be interpreted as sexual, or may not be enjoyed (despite sexual interpretation)(54). Even a frankly dysphoric emotional response may occur. Throbbing and tingling and feelings of urgency for more genital contact and vaginal entry occur less consistently in sexually healthy women than do the equivalent sensations in men. Sexually healthy women typically experience these confirmatory sexual stimuli indirectly by the enjoyment of manual or oral stimulation or genital stimulation with a vibrator, which are all enhanced when vulval engorgement occurs.

It is important to note that qualitative research has shown that many women cannot clearly distinguish between desire and arousal (55). Some women refer to genital and nongenital physical sensations as components of their desire; this is especially true of younger women. Investigators have found that in sexually healthy women, a highly variable correlation exists between objective measurement of genital congestion (as measured with the vaginal plethysmograph) and subjective arousal (56–58). The measurement most commonly used for vaginal congestion is the vaginal pulse amplitude, which represents the phasic change in congestion with each heartbeat. To examine arousal, women view a neutral film followed by an erotic film, and the percentage of increase in vaginal pulse amplitude is noted along with their ratings of subjective arousal. Most women with sexual arousal disorder who have been studied during the past 30 years show increases in vaginal pulse amplitude in response to visual erotica similar to those of sexually healthy women (56, 58). However, these women mostly report minimal or absent sexual arousal during erotic films, and they may report negative emotions. Functional brain imaging of women's arousal as they view erotic videos does not show significant association between brain activation patterns and vaginal pulse amplitude; this is true for women with and without desire and arousal deficit (59). Similarly, in such women, awareness of genital sensations is minimal, correlating poorly with objective measurement of congestion in response to erotic stimuli.

The genital response appears to be a reflex automatic entity that can be elicited in response to a stimulus that is deemed simply sexual and not erotic or potentially arousing; eg, viewing a video of primates engaged in mating (57). The degree of congestion of their extensive clitoral structures and vaginal circulation is not accurately perceived by women; it is clear that women's arousal cannot be measured by their report of genital swelling lubrication response. Recommended definitions of disordered arousal include the different components of arousal—genital and subjective excitement (56). The final *DSM-5* definition includes a potential loss of genital sexual sensitivity (53).

Whereas genital arousal is a reflex, rapid in onset, subjective arousal is a slow process and documented to be strongly modulated by cognitions and emotions. An important inhibitory factor with strong empiric support is "arousal contingency" (for example, "When I am getting aroused, the slightest thing can turn me off.") (60). The type of stimulation, the context, her ability to attend (61), the number of distractions and disengaging thoughts, including fear of negative outcome (62, 63), concurrent emotions, including joy and affirmation or, alternatively, anxiety and shame (64, 65) are all known to modulate a woman's experience of arousal moment by moment. Research identified more early maladaptive schemas (described as stable, enduring themes that build up during childhood and develop throughout life to influence the processing of adult experiences) in women with sexual dysfunctions (66). When arousal does follow, and the stimulation continues for a sufficient length of time, its intensity can increase and trigger desire; at that point her focus becomes her need of sexual satisfaction. The latter may or may not include orgasm but usually requires freedom from any pain, partner dysfunction (67), or negative emotional conclusion. Positive experiences reinforce subsequent sexual motivation. The cycle shown in Figure 1 may be repeated many times during one encounter. This cyclicity and phase overlap predict the well-documented comorbidity of desire and arousal disorders (8, 68).

The focus on the mind's processing of stimuli is in keeping with Janssen's information processing model (69) and also with the concept of sexual excitation versus sexual inhibition as explored by Sanders and Graham (60). Thus, the circular model depicted in Figure 1 is composite and also allows for the marked variability of response for any given woman and among different women who consider their sexual lives to be rewarding and functional.

Sexual Orientation

Similar to the concept of diversity in sexual response cycles, sexual orientation reflects a continuum of same-sex attraction. Studies confirm that many people experience at least occasional same-sex attraction, far fewer act on it, and even fewer identify as gay (70). Women's sexuality is described as "fluid," which means that orientation may change (71). Terms, such as "mostly straight" and "bi-curious" are increasingly used. A transition from lesbian to bisexual is common (and such women refer to themselves as "wasbians" or "hasbians"). Female same-sex sexuality differs in many ways from male same-sex sexuality (72)—women may experience more discrepancies between sexual attraction and sexual behavior; a late and abrupt onset of same-sex sexuality (often after a heterosexual marriage), and increased fluctuations in their sexual identity and behavior over time. A web-based survey of 1,784 individuals supported a five-category classification: 1) heterosexual, 2) mostly heterosexual, 3) bisexual, 4) mostly gay and mostly lesbian, and 5) gay and lesbian. These five groups differed in partnerships and attraction in a manner reflecting a continuous distribution of sexual orientation (73).

Sexual Identity

Current loosening of a two-sex system allows the diversity of sex to be acknowledged. The spectrum includes biologic men who take feminizing hormones, dress as women but retain their penises, and are referred to as "he/she's" and lesbians who identify as male and dress and conduct themselves as male but take no masculinizing hormones and do not consider reassignment surgery, often calling themselves "bois." The latter clearly require gynecologic care similar to nontranssexual women.

Gynecologists may be involved in the care of transsexual men (female to male) by performing elective hysterectomy and bilateral oophorectomy as part of initial gender reassignment surgery. Also, if hysterectomy is not undertaken, endometrial effects of long-term testosterone treatment need to be monitored. Gynecologists also may be involved in puberty suppression to allow adolescent women with gender dysphoria to explore the disorder and contemplate reassignment surgery without the distress from the physical changes of puberty.

Basic Science Update

Examples within sexual and nonsexual physiology illustrate biologic sequelae of psychologic factors. For example, psychologic stress is known to be associated with changes in the hypothalamic–pituitary–adrenal and hypothalamic–pituitary–gonadal axes, the immune system, and even with neuronal (hippocampal) atrophy or regeneration. The most common form of chronic dyspareunia, provoked vestibulodynia, is associated with abnormal proliferation of free nerve endings, accumulation of chronic inflammatory cells, and increased levels of cytokines in the involved areas of skin. Moreover, pain thresholds elsewhere in the bodies of the affected individuals are lower than those of unaffected individuals, which indicate widespread changes to pain pathways. Robust evidence shows increased stress in women with provoked vestibulodynia (74). Thus, it would appear that stress plus certain personality traits that may be associated with increased sensitivity to stress predispose some individuals to developing and maintaining provoked vestibulodynia (75).

Central Sexual Neurophysiology

Although knowledge of the neurobiology of sexual desire and response is incomplete, multiple neurotransmitters, peptides, and hormones are known to be involved. Noradrenaline, dopamine, melanocortin, oxytocin, and serotonin that activates 5HT receptors 1A and 2C are prosexual; prolactin, serotonin that activates other receptors, and γ-aminobutyric acid (GABA), are inhibitory. Functional brain imaging suggests that sexual arousal involves complex brain circuitry that links cortical limbic and paralimbic regions that are associated with cognition, attention, motivation, and emotions and also the autonomic nervous system through the hypothalamus (76). Activation in the hypothalamus does not correlate strongly with subjective arousal in women (although it does in similar studies in men), which echoes the poor correlation between women's subjective arousal and their measured genital response. Disease states give clues to the underlying central biology, eg, reduced sexual desire with hyperprolactinemia, hypothyroidism, and hypopituitary disorder. Hormone levels can be measured during the sexual response, but these findings may reflect the consequence of sexual outcome rather than the cause, eg, increased oxytocin levels with arousal and increased prolactin levels after orgasm. The value of blood level measurement as opposed to cerebrospinal fluid level measurement is highly questionable.

Animal studies show that not only can dopamine and other compounds replicate the increase in sexual behavior mediated by the progesterone receptors in the rodent hypothalamus, but that environmental influence (presence of a male animal) can afford exactly the same change in sexual behavior (77, 78). Thus, the social environmental factors can cause ligand-independent activation of sex hormone receptors. Possible human analogies include the increased arousability in some women (without depression) who were given a dopaminergic drug (bupropion) (79); the increased arousability also was achieved by acquiring a new partner (80). Thus, a complex interplay exists between the neurotransmitters, peptides, and sex hormones and between environmental and neuroendocrine factors.

Peripheral Sexual Neurophysiology

Vulval genital congestion involves the active neurogenic dilation of sinusoidal blood spaces in the extensive corporal clitoral tissue; the glans, shaft, rami, bulbs, and periurethral components comprise approximately 40 cubic centimeters of vascular tissue (Fig. 2). In a small number of women, an area of erotic sensitivity exists in the anterior vaginal wall. No scientific consensus exists regarding the any actual structure or "G spot." However, the female urethra is surrounded by glandular tissue that may swell with increased secretions during arousal. The gland ducts typically feed into the urethra, but some evidence also exists of paraurethral ducts that open into the urethral meatus. This may account for the possibility of so-called female ejaculation at orgasm. The glandular fluid contains acid phosphatase, which distinguishes it from urine.

Exactly how much disruption to the autonomic plexus between the vagina and bladder can occur without a negative effect on vulvar congestion is unclear—radical hysterectomy for cancer of the cervix interferes with vaginal engorgement to such an extent that, despite taking estrogen therapy, patients have persistent

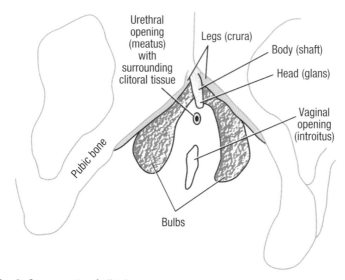

Fig. 2. Components of clitoris.

dryness and dyspareunia (81). Midurethral slings for urinary incontinence may disrupt autonomic innervation of the vulva (82). Vulvar structures engorge but do not become erect. The tunica is thinner than penile tunica and trapping of venous blood does not occur, but instead blood pools with some persistent inflow and outflow. Nitric oxide is a major neurotransmitter and acts through various mechanisms, including the activation of cyclic guanosine monophosphate to relax smooth muscle.

Vasoactive intestinal polypeptide (VIP), peptide histidine methionine, helospectin, neuropeptide Y, substance P, and calcitonin gene-related peptide also play a role. Vaginal congestion mostly is effected by VIP, which induces smooth muscle relaxation through cyclic adenosine monophosphate and is downgraded by neutral and soluble endopeptidases. With vaginal arterial dilation, blood flow to the submucosal vaginal capillaries increases, which in turns results in increased interstitial fluid production. Interstitial fluid diffuses more quickly across the vaginal epithelial cells and onto the lumen so the lubrication fluid in the aroused state contains less potassium and more sodium than in the nonaroused state. How important the contribution of permeability of the epithelial cells is to the process of lubrication is currently unclear. Small nerve fibres that contain calcitonin gene-related peptide end directly on epithelial cells, which possibly modulates their permeability. Relaxation of the vaginal wall smooth muscle that enables the vagina to move up into the pelvis is likely mediated by VIP (83).

Detumescence of clitoral tissue and reduction of blood flow through vaginal capillaries (resulting in reduction of lubrication and maintenance of vaginal nonvascular smooth muscle tone) is thought to be caused predominantly by noradrenaline that is released from adrenergic nerves acting on α1-adrenergic receptors. However, the calcium ion (Ca^{2+})-sensitizing RhoA–Rho kinase pathway may be involved.

The genital arousal response involves sympathetic and parasympathetic nerves. Traditional markers of increased sympathetic nerve activity, such as elevated heart rate, blood pressure, and respiratory rate, accompany sexual arousal. Pelvic sympathetic postganglionic neurons primarily release noradrenaline and adenosine triphosphate, but some neurones that are involved in vulval congestion release acetylcholine, nitric oxide, and VIP. Input from the ganglia of the caudal sympathetic chain that contains noradrenaline and likely neuropeptide Y produce the expected vasoconstriction. Input from the hypogastric nerve (also sympathetic) that passes through ganglionic relay stations in the pelvic plexus can produce vasodilation and vulval congestion as well as the opposite effect. Parasympathetic nerves S-2 through S-4 release nitric oxide, which mediates vasodilation, and acetylcholine, which acts prejunctionally or postjunctionally by blocking noradrenergic vasoconstrictor mechanisms and by stimulating the endothelium to release nitric oxide.

An increase in sympathetic tone as from exercise, hyperventilation, or ephedrine increases the physiologic genital arousal response. Similarly, the presence of anxiety-provoking visual stimuli increases the genital physiologic congestive response to subsequent erotic visual cues. Heightened sympathetic activity accompanies many emotions, including fear, and the excitement that accompanies knowledge that something pleasant is about to happen. Also, it is associated with the state of sexual arousal.

The neurobiology of orgasm is poorly understood. Although nerve damage to autonomic nerves between the vagina and bladder reduces genital congestion, it does not preclude orgasm, for example from a vibrator placed on the mons pubis. However, this does not necessarily mean orgasm is conveyed by somatic pudendal nerve fibers because the pudendal nerve also carries sympathetic fibers. The sexual sensitivity of genital structures has received little attention. Nerve terminals in the glans clitoris, known as corpuscular receptors, are thought to be involved. These are mechanoreceptors; their density is variable but can be 14-fold greater than the density of similar receptors on the glans penis (84). Immunohistologic studies have identified calcitonin gene-related peptide and substance P likely allowing touch and pain sensations.

The Roles of Sex Hormones in Sexual Response

Levels of estrogen fluctuate premenopausally throughout the menstrual cycle and appear to be adequate for sexual response. After menopause, the estrogen levels detected in the blood reflect estrogen activity to a limited degree only—estrogen is produced outside the ovary and functions as a paracrine or intracrine factor. The estrogen in the blood has "spilled over" after intracellular production from adrenal precursor hormones (Fig. 3). Compared with women with low body mass index, women with high body mass index have higher estrogen levels related to increased numbers of adipose cells and increased aromatization and activity of cytochrome P450.

ESTROGEN

Estrogen is known to affect mood and sleep so its central action may indirectly influence sexual response. A high number of estrogen receptors are present in the smooth muscle, endothelium, and

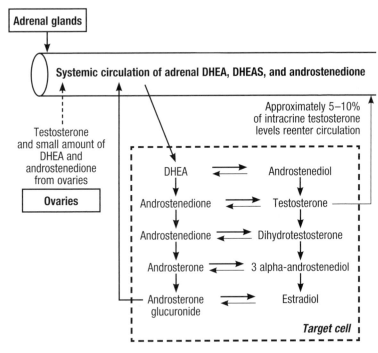

Fig. 3. Intracrine production of testosterone in target cell from circulating precursor dehydroepiandrosterone. Other precursor hormones include androstene-3β,17β-diol, androstenedione, and dehydroepiandrosterone sulfate. Only approximately 5–10% of intracrine testosterone levels enter circulation. Intracrine testosterone is further metabolized, mainly to androsterone glucuronide, which diffuses into the circulation and can be measured. Abbreviations: DHEA indicates dehydroepiandrosterone; DHEAS, dehydroepiandrosterone sulfate.

epithelium of the vagina, vestibule, and labia. The number of vessels decreases with estrogen lack; the pallor of vulval atrophy frequently is marked. Also changed is the extracellular matrix, hence collagen and elastin interact with proteoglycans to form a dense tissue that has decreased flexibility. Loss, shortening, and narrowing of vaginal rugae can occur. All these changes contribute to pain not only with sexual intercourse or penetration with fingers or dildo, but sometimes also with manual stimulation of vulval structures. Some postmenopausal women describe loss of swelling of vulval structures associated with their loss of genital response. Others suggest they have never actually been aware of swelling, but simply report no pleasure from direct genital stimulation.

The roles of nitric oxide and VIP in genital congestion highlight the significance of estrogen for adequate lubrication. The biologic activity of nitric oxide is increased by an estrogen receptor-mediated antioxidant effect. Endothelial function in nongenital areas is impaired in postmenopausal women. Estrogen therapy is associated with upregulation of estrogen receptors on the vessel wall. Vasoactive intestinal polypeptide also requires a minimum of estrogen for its activity. The limited investigation of neurotransmitters involved in vaginal tissues suggests that, in postmenopausal women, VIP level is markedly reduced as is nitric oxide synthase level. However, despite the major decrease in estrogen activity after menopause, dyspareunia from vulvovaginal atrophy is not universal. One study suggests that when intracrine production allows serum levels to exceed 20 pmol/L, pain is less common (85). Symptoms of pain and signs of atrophy do not necessarily correlate. The matter is complex; psychophysiologic studies to date suggest that the increase in vaginal congestion associated with a sexual stimulus is similar in women with estrogen repletion and women with estrogen deficiency (86). Small magnetic resonance imaging (MRI) studies suggest a similar increase in clitoral volume in response to arousing erotic stimuli in premenopausal women compared with postmenopausal women (87). However, such studies do not measure absolute levels of blood flow but relative increases in congestion over baseline. A study of 300 North American women consecutively examined within 12 months of discontinuing estrogen therapy found that 290 of these women showed signs of vaginal atrophy accompanied by increased local pH levels (88). More research is needed to understand why only some women are sexually symptomatic, but evidence is accruing to confirm the importance of psychologic factors (89). Based on animal data, hyperalgesia caused by proliferation of nociceptors caused by hyperalgesia can follow estrogen deficit (90). This information emphasizes that prescribing a simple lubricant may not restore the health of atrophic vaginal tissues. Estrogen supplementation may be needed for painless intercourse or other sexual vaginal penetration. Continued sexual activity may be helpful (91), but not sufficient, to maintain vascularity, intercellular space resistance (92), and the activity of many genes governing growth factors, immune factors, and interleukins, all of which require estrogen (93). In one large survey, despite continuing to be sexually active, approximately 60% of postmenopausal women experienced symptoms of atrophy (3).

Urinary frequency and urgency may be related to changes from estrogen lack, including atrophy of the bladder trigone, decreased sensitivity of α-adrenergic receptors in the bladder neck and urethral sphincter, and thinning of the urethral mucosa and surrounding connective tissue. The urethra and trigone have high numbers of estrogen receptors. Sexual consequences include avoiding orgasms for fear of incontinence and discomfort from massaging the anterior vaginal wall—possibly a former site of intense pleasure from the stimulation of engorging spongiosal tissue around the urethra. The increased pH and altered vaginal flora from predominantly gram-negative organisms that are associated with estrogen lack may predispose women to urinary tract infections, decreasing their motivation to be sexual. They also may be associated with dyspareunia. Some reviews conclude that local estrogen application may help urgency, frequency, and incontinence from overactive bladder to a modest degree but long-term management was unclear. In contrast, systemic estrogen may worsen symptoms (94, 95).

ANDROGENS

In men, serum levels of testosterone well below the lower limit of normal are associated with loss of sexual desire along with loss of nocturnal erections, volume of ejaculate, and delay in orgasm.

Therefore, it is reasonable to consider whether testosterone lack in women modulates their sexual desire and function. However, the sound scientific evidence is lacking. Serum levels of testosterone do not correlate with women's sexual function according to large epidemiologic studies (96, 97). Two confounding factors were thought to have precluded showing an association between low testosterone and women's sexual dysfunction. The first factor involved a difficulty with available assays that were originally designed to measure male range of testosterone. When a more sensitive standard assay, involving mass spectrometry, was used in a study of 121 women with low initial desire and low subjective arousal and 124 women in a control group, researchers found no group difference in terms of measured serum testosterone levels (98). The second confounding factor was associated with the lack of means to measure intracrine testosterone levels until the past decade. Studies have now shown a presence of wide range in androgen metabolites—most notably androsterone glucuronide— among women of any given age group (99). These metabolites reflect the total androgen activity, ie, ovarian plus intracrine (Fig. 3). The expected decrease in androgen metabolites with age has been confirmed (98, 99). More recently, androsterone glucuronide levels were compared in 121 women with low desire and 124 women without low desire, and no group differences were found (98).

Reduction of Testosterone Production with Age. Ovarian and intracrine sources of testosterone are important contributors to the total testosterone activity in women. The adrenal glands are the major source of precursor hormones dehydroepiandrosterone (DHEA), dehydroepiandrosterone sulfate (DHEAS), androstenedione, and 5-androstene-3β, 17β-diol. Their levels decrease with age by approximately two thirds between age 30 years and age 70 years (99, 100). After natural menopause, ovarian testosterone production continues to a variable extent and ovarian production of androstenedione and DHEA, both of which can be converted in peripheral cells to testosterone and estrogen, is reduced. Aging is associated with decreasing sexual desire. However, this decrease is not associated with an increased prevalence of the disorder because distress is absent (101). The former hypoactive sexual desire disorder (as per *DSM-IV-TR*) and the current

sexual interest/arousal disorder (as per *DSM-5*) are characterized by deficiency or absence of sexual fantasies and interest/
arousal for sexual activity (and in *DSM-5*, by decreased pleasure,
receptivity, and initiation) that causes marked distress (53).
Similar total androgen activity has been reported in women with
hypoactive sexual desire disorder and without hypoactive sexual
desire disorder (98).

Sexual Desire After Surgical Menopause. In contrast to natural
menopause that has little effect on intracrine or ovarian testosterone production, surgical menopause obviously removes all
ovarian testosterone, ovarian DHEA, and androstenedione production. Some cross-sectional epidemiologic data from studies
of women with hypoactive sexual desire disorder show that
surgically menopausal women are distressed by decreased desire
more than age-matched women with intact ovaries (42, 43).
However, they do not have a higher prevalence of low desire
per se (16). A recent study of 1,352 women showed no difference in the report of sexual ideation, sexual function, or sexual
problems between women who have had and women who have
not had bilateral oophorectomy (102). Moreover, prospective
studies of elective bilateral salpingo-oophorectomy along with
a needed elective perimenopausal hysterectomy do not identify
any decrease in sexual function in women monitored for up to
3 years (44, 45). However, in some instances of nonelective surgery, the thematic context of bilateral oophorectomy is likely to
impair sexual desire and function, for example, in women who
were treated for malignant disease or those who desired to pre-
serve their fertility.

Testosterone in the Brain—Neurosteroids. It remains possible
that testosterone modulates desire and response, but that the
systemic production or deficit is of little relevance. Testosterone
is produced de novo within the central nervous system (CNS)
from cholesterol (103). This production appears to be quite
widespread within the CNS. Adaptive changes to reductions
in serum levels of sex hormones associated with age and with
menopause occur in the brain; steroidogenic enzymes and sex
receptors are upregulated (104). How any supplemental testosterone might affect neurosteroid production is not known.

Dehydroepiandrosterone also is a neurosteroid. In addition to being a precursor of androgens and estrogen, DHEA has many other functions that involve membrane receptors. Pathways include activation of nitric oxide synthase and modulation of GABA receptors and σ receptors. Studies have not shown systemic DHEA in a physiologic dosage to improve sexual desire or function (105). In one small study, postmenopausal women with nonsexual climacteric symptoms chose HT or vitamin D supplementation. Those who chose HT were further randomized to receive estrogen and progesterone, tibolone, or 10 mg of DHEA. All three HT regimens resulted in improved menopausal symptoms and scores on the sexuality questionnaire (106).

Androgen Receptor Sensitivity. A length polymorphism in a repeated sequence of the androgen receptor gene has been known to modulate the activity of the androgen receptor. However, the molecular structure of the androgen receptor in women with sexual disorders and without sexual disorders has not been studied. Variability in numbers and activities of the cofactors for the androgen receptor further clouds the issue. It should be noted that women with complete androgen insufficiency may not report sexual dysfunction or lack of sexual desire (107, 108).

Transdermal Testosterone Trials. Two pharmaceutical companies have conducted randomized controlled trials (RCTs) of transdermal testosterone supplementation that involved women who reported reduced initial or anticipatory desire. These studies yielded conflicting results. No trials studied women who lack anticipatory desire and the ability to become aroused to trigger desire during the sexual encounter.

The first series of RCTs used matrix patches to increase testosterone levels to the high premenopausal range in medically and mentally healthy postmenopausal women who reported loss of desire since menopause but were still able to be aroused and have satisfying sexual encounters approximately two to three times per month before any therapy was given. Four studies involved surgically menopausal women who took estrogen therapy (109–112). The first trial found that 300 micrograms, but not 150 micrograms or 450 micrograms, of transdermal testosterone daily significantly increased the frequency of sexually satisfying events (P=.049) compared with placebo. Combined results from all four studies indicated that sexually satisfying experiences increased to approximately five per month with active drug and four per month with placebo. Data pooled from an unpublished validated questionnaire showed that scores in the desire and arousal scales were significantly increased when active drug was administered in the first three studies. The fourth smaller study recruited women who were prescribed transdermal estrogen and showed a significant increase in desire and response scales but not in the number of sexually satisfying events (112).

A second pharmaceutical company released results from its two phase III transdermal (gel) testosterone studies of 1,172 postmenopausal women; one half of these women received systemic estrogen (113). Published details are limited, but recruited women appear similar to those in the testosterone patch studies, and similar serum levels of testosterone were achieved. Neither endpoint, namely an increase in number of satisfying sexual encounters or an increase in mean sexual desire, significantly differed from placebo in either study (114).

The testosterone patch studies also involved 549 naturally menopausal women who took HT who were able to have sexually satisfying events at least twice per month. Those who received 300 micrograms of testosterone showed a statistically significant increase in satisfying sexual events and desire and response scales compared with placebo (115). Total testosterone levels exceeded the normal range for premenopausal women, at least in part caused by increased levels of sex hormone-binding globulin associated with the concurrent oral estrogen therapy.

Two studies of the 300-microgram testosterone patch involved women with estrogen deficiency. One study recruited 814 participants and showed a significant increase in satisfying sexual events in the naturally menopausal women from the active drug but not in the small subgroup of surgically menopausal women (116). Only 464 participants completed treatment with similar distribution of high discontinuation rates in all three arms. A second study of 272 naturally menopausal women showed a significant increase in satisfying sexual events. A total of 73% of the participants were not receiving systemic estrogen therapy (117).

A previous small study had shown minimal or no benefit from transdermal testosterone in women with estrogen deficiency with a history of cancer (118).

Supplementing testosterone, but not estrogen, is nonphysiologic. Postmenopausal women already have high testosterone-to-estrogen ratios compared with premenopausal women. Long-term sequelae of accentuating the altered testosterone-to-estrogen ratio are unknown. Endogenously high testosterone along with obesity in older women is associated with insulin resistance and increased cardiovascular (CV) morbidity (119). Moreover, aromatization of exogenous testosterone to estrogen is likely, and initiating systemic estrogen supplementation 10 years after menopause is known to increase cardiovascular risk.

Minimal benefit was reported from transdermal testosterone given to 261 premenopausal women (120). Just one of three doses aimed to increase free testosterone levels to the high normal range for premenopausal women showed a statistically significant benefit at 16 weeks; the middle dose (90 microliters daily) increased the number of satisfying sexual events by a mean of 0.8 in the previous month. No doses were associated with any improvement beyond placebo in sexual function and satisfaction scales.

The criteria for recruitment to trials of testosterone are problematic; it is not certain that the recruited women had any sexual disorder, and the focus has been consistently on the frequency of satisfying events in women able to have such experiences. When clarified, it is apparent that approximately 50% of experiences reported by women were satisfactory at baseline (116). Therefore, women did not have consistent dysfunction, which refutes a biologic cause or a need for a biologic remedy and instead supports psychologic, relationship, or contextual factors that are inherently variable. An improvement was reported in the secondary endpoints of desire and response subscales in the questionnaires, but increasing the degree of pleasure and arousal currently experienced may not necessarily imply that absent pleasure and absent arousal would be remedied. Tibolone with its androgenic, estrogenic, and progestogenic properties was shown repeatedly to increase desire and response scores in sexually functional women recruited for nonsexual reasons for postmenopausal HT, and yet the more recent RCT of sexually dysfunctional women showed benefit only comparable with that afforded by transdermal estradiol and norethisterone acetate (121).

Even when carefully excluding women with clinical depression, a higher number of depressed and anxious thoughts, more mood lability, and low self-image are noted by women who report desire concerns (7). Is it possible that women without these characteristics would not be distressed to have approximately three satisfactory sexual experiences per month, and would an increase to five rather than four such events be important to them? The documented benefit of testosterone on mood may be relevant.

Blinding of testosterone therapy trials is difficult because facial hair growth often is a very private concern, which is remedied by plucking and is not reported. The lack of demonstrated androgen deficit in women with hypoactive sexual desire disorder, with or without arousal disorder, must be kept in mind (98).

Long-term safety issues of combined testosterone and estrogen add to those of estrogen alone. Trials typically do not provide data beyond 2–3 years of study; a planned 5-year safety study of testosterone gel (which proved equal to placebo in benefit) in women older than 50 years of age with at least two cardiovascular risk factors, endorsed by the U.S. Food and Drug Administration (FDA), has been discontinued. The reason given is that stopping now will save costs and already 3,200 and 1,700 women have been monitored for 1 year and 2 years, respectively (122). Neither excess cardiovascular events nor breast cancer were reported in the active arm according to an unblinded independent Data Monitoring Committee (123). Most patch studies were of 6-month duration, but researchers report that open label extensions provided safety data to 2 years and caution that the usual 6-month duration and relatively small number of participants limit the ability to detect CV signals (124). No clinically relevant changes in liver function, carbohydrate metabolism, lipid levels, clotting parameters, or hematology were noted (124). The number of women involved is unclear. A concern has been raised that the target high-normal serum concentrations of testosterone and dehydrotestosterone were exceeded in a significant number of the women in the patch studies (125). Indirect data support risk increase and decrease for breast cancer from testosterone supplementation. One review concludes that the available clinical literature does not permit conclusions on safety (126).

Cardiovascular safety remains of concern. Unlike men, women with high endogenous testosterone levels are more likely to develop insulin resistance and CV risk (119, 127), but how this relates to postmenopausal testosterone therapy is unknown. Currently, long-term estrogen therapy is not advocated. Women who begin estrogen therapy at menopause may show CV benefit rather than harm, but no evidence exists that after 10–15 years of exogenous estrogen therapy the endothelial function remains sufficiently healthy to allow its indefinite prescription. However, a woman's sexual life tends to continue as long as she has a sexually active partner. Thus, the long-term safety of estrogen and testosterone supplementation is a crucial topic. The Endocrine Society advised against testosterone supplementation for women (45), and these recommendations were similar to European recommendations (128). An in-press updated guideline from The Endocrine Society, citing a meta-analysis that included only the published randomized trials of testosterone (129), suggests a 3–6 month trial of high physiologic dose testosterone therapy strictly limited to women with hypoactive sexual desire disorder (as per *DSM-IV-TR*) after careful diagnosis. The 300-microgram testosterone patch was licensed in Europe for hypoactive sexual desire disorder associated with surgical menopause in women who take estrogen therapy, but it is not recommended for naturally menopausal women or those who use conjugated estrogens. The cited cause for these restrictions is a lack of established safety beyond 1 year. Currently, no approved testosterone formulation exists for women. The Marketing Authorization Holder responsible for Intrinsa, Warner Chilcott UK Ltd, notified the European Commission in March 2012 of its decision to voluntarily withdraw the marketing authorization for Intrinsa for commercial reasons (130).

Intravaginal Testosterone. It was shown that local delivery of the main precursor hormone, namely DHEA, into the vagina may not only efficiently treat typical symptoms of vulvar vaginal atrophy associated with estrogen deficiency but it restores genital sexual sensitivity so that orgasms are more easily reached and more intense (131). This therapy appeared to be truly local without any increase in serum estrogen or testosterone or in their metabolites (132). Further study is needed to confirm these results. The desire, as rated on the questionnaire used in the study, also improved significantly with the use of intravaginal testosterone, compared with placebo. This may reflect increased awareness of genital congestion or increased sexual motivation. Restored vaginal lubrication, coital comfort, and easier and more intense orgasms could certainly improve motivation. The systemic absorption of DHEA was small; levels remained in the range of older women (132).

A comparative study that involved administration of twice-weekly vaginal 2% testosterone (0.5 mg) with conjugated equine estrogen (0.625 mg) showed more sexual benefit than the administration of estrogen alone (133). Serum testosterone levels increased to values within the normal postmenopausal range.

Classification of Sexual Disorders

International Classification of Diseases-10

Uncertainty exists as to what exactly constitutes a sexual disorder. Clearly, this is not simply a medical matter—what is considered "disordered" varies with time and culture. The World Health Organization's International Classification of Diseases-10 (ICD-10) suggests sexual dysfunctions are "the various ways in which an individual is unable to participate in a sexual relationship as he or she would wish" (134). The ICD-10 is in the process of revision, with new definitions expected in 2015.

Diagnostic and Statistical Manual of Mental Disorders, Fifth Edition

The American Psychiatric Association's *DSM-5* suggests sexual dysfunctions are "a heterogeneous group of disorders that are typically characterized by a clinically significant disturbance in a person's ability to respond to sexually or to experience sexual pleasure. Aging may be associated with a normative decrease in sexual response. The latter has biological underpinning, yet is usually experienced in an intrapersonal, interpersonal, and cultural context" (53). The *DSM-5* was published in 2013, superseding the *DSM-IV-TR*, which was published in 2000. The changes incorporated in *DSM-5* indicate that women's sexual response and problems associated with it will no longer simply follow a male model given the sound empirical and qualitative study to support a nonlinear, highly variable response cycle of overlapping phases of variable order. Thus, the *DSM-5* classifications of disorders of female hypoactive sexual desire disorder, female sexual arousal disorder, and female orgasmic disorder (mirroring male hypoactive sexual desire disorder, erectile dysfunction, and male orgasmic disorder) are replaced by three categories: 1) female sexual interest/arousal disorder; 2) female orgasmic disorder; and 3) genitopelvic pain/penetration disorder (given the overlap between vaginismus and dyspareunia). Evaluation and management sections of this monograph will follow these *DSM-5* definitions of sexual dysfunction. Sexual aversion disorder is no longer listed. This may be in part because "aversive" responses to genital touch are commonly present in women with vaginismus or genitopelvic pain/penetration disorder. A global aversion to anything sexual may be better understood as a phobia. For all disorders, specifiers are proposed as shown in Box 5.

A distress criterion is included in *DSM-IV-TR* and *DSM-5*. Although distress avoids the overdiagnosis of a condition in a woman whose sexual response is satisfying to her, but would otherwise merit a diagnosis of sexual disorder, it is unusual in medicine to base a diagnosis only in the presence of personal distress. For example, a woman still has diabetes even if she has no distress about its presence or even if she is totally unaware of its presence. Furthermore, the difficulty remains that if the partner is distressed (for example, by the woman's nonorgasmic response), the resulting interpersonal difficulties can cause the woman distress thereby categorizing her sexual function as disordered. Insisting on distress, for inclusion of women into clinical trials is proving to be problematic. When the question of distress is discussed, a typical reply is: "Although I am here for help and I am very motivated, I am not personally distressed. Although I have lost desire, in a way, it is not an issue, but I am distressed at the thought of what this may do to my marriage. I am distressed on an intellectual rather than an emotional level." Only a subgroup of women with absent sexual desire continue to yearn for their former desire and "want to want" sex.

Box 5. Revisions to the American Psychiatric Association's Classification of Sexual Disorders

Disorder is diagnosed only if clinically significant distress or impairment is present. Disorders are identified as early-onset (lifelong) versus late-onset (acquired). The sexual dysfunction is not better explained by a nonsexual psychiatric disorder; by the effects of a substance (eg, a drug of abuse or a medication); by a medical condition; or by relationship distress, partner violence, or other significant stressors.

Female Sexual Interest/Arousal Disorder

Lack of sexual interest or arousal for a minimum duration of 6 months as manifested by at least three of the following factors:

1. Absent/reduced interest in sexual activity

2. Absent/reduced sexual/erotic thoughts or fantasies

3. Absent/reduced sexual excitement/pleasure during sexual activity and typically unreceptive to a partner's attempts to initiate sexual activity

4. Absent/reduced sexual interest/pleasure during sexual activity in all or almost all (approximately 75–100%) sexual encounters

5. Absent/reduced sexual interest/arousal in response to any internal or external sexual/erotic cues (eg, written, verbal, and visual)

6. Absent/reduced genital or nongenital sensations during sexual activity on all or almost all (approximately 75–100%) sexual encounters

(continued)

Box 5. Revisions to the American Psychiatric Association's Classification of Sexual Disorders (continued)

Female Orgasmic Disorder

At least one of the two following symptoms where the symptom must have been present for a minimum duration of approximately 6 months and be experienced on all or almost all (approximately 75%) occasions of sexual activity:

1. Marked delay in, marked infrequency of, or absence of orgasm
2. Markedly reduced intensity of orgasmic sensation

Genitopelvic Pain/Penetration Disorder

Persistent or recurrent difficulties for a minimum duration of approximately 6 months with one or more of the following factors:

1. Marked difficulty with vaginal intercourse or penetration
2. Marked vulvovaginal or pelvic pain during attempts of vaginal intercourse or penetration attempts
3. Marked fear or anxiety regarding either vulvovaginal or pelvic pain on vaginal penetration
4. Marked tensing or tightening of the pelvic floor muscles during attempted vaginal penetration

The merging of former terms "vaginismus" and "dyspareunia" has some merit. Although some women report typical phobic avoidance of penetration such that penile introital contact has never been possible, and physical examination has to be deferred until therapy enables it to be performed, often the condition is complicated. For example, the woman gives a history of phobic avoidance and fear, subsequent examination confirms vaginistic reaction, but once therapy allows a careful detailed introital examination, allodynia of the vestibule is confirmed, thus diagnosing "vaginismus by history," but current provoked vestibulodynia on examination.

Screening

Box 6 outlines examples of how to establish a dialogue regarding sexual function when the woman is presenting with nonsexual concerns. Respectful careful listening will not only clarify the problems but is in itself therapeutic.

 Box 6. Establishing a Dialogue

Background Considerations

- When inquiring about sexual difficulties, avoiding preconceptions about what is "normal" or "abnormal" and accepting diversity and variation will allow women to disclose problems.

- Using gender-neutral language and not assuming heterosexual orientation is important; for example, a pregnant woman may have a female partner.

- It is necessary to realize that women's sexuality is "fluid"; for example, self-labeling from lesbian to bisexual or heterosexual over a 5-year period is not uncommon.

- Sexual identification, attraction, and behavior may not all match. It is important to ask in a sensitive manner about contact with men and women when problems are being assessed.

Screening for Sexual Dysfunction and Initiating Discussion When Sex Is Not the Presenting Concern

- Before performing surgical procedures or prescribing medications or hormone therapy, ask the patient: "Your surgery or medication is not expected to interfere with your sexual function. Do you presently have any difficulties with sexual desire, arousal, or enjoyment, or do you have any pain?"

(continued)

Box 6. Establishing a Dialogue *(continued)*

- During a routine antenatal visit, ask the patient: "Women's sexual needs can change during pregnancy or after delivery. Do you have any problems or questions now? No evidence exists that intercourse or orgasm leads to miscarriage. Any bleeding or spotting requires checking and postponing sexual activity until evaluated completely. Often, fatigue and nausea will limit sexual interest in the first 3 months, but then your usual sexual feelings will likely return. Toward the end of pregnancy most women are not very interested in sex."

- During a complicated antenatal visit, ask the patient about present concerns and specify the specific restrictions that are needed (eg, no orgasm and no intercourse or other penetrative activity).

- After one or more pregnancy losses, encourage the patient by saying: "Some women temporarily lose desire for sex after a miscarriage. This is normal. Couples often concentrate on affectionate touching while they both grieve. Allow yourselves some time to recover. If sexual problems persist, they can be addressed."

- During infertility treatment, encourage the patient by saying: "All this testing and timed intercourse (or inseminations) and disappointments plus the financial burdens can add stress to your sex life. Try to make time to be intimate just for pleasure, not to conceive. If you experience sexual problems that persist, they can be addressed."

- During the postpartum period, encourage the patient by saying: "It may be some weeks or months before you have the energy for sex, especially if your sleep remains interrupted. This is normal. If sexual problems persist or if you have pain, this can be addressed."

(continued)

Box 6. Establishing a Dialogue *(continued)*

- During perimenopause or after menopause, explain to the patient: "Many women have rewarding sex after menopause because they do not need to be concerned by birth control issues, and they have more privacy. If you find the opposite or you begin to have pain or cannot become aroused, these things can be addressed. Do you have any concerns now?"

- When a patient has depression, explain to her: "Studies suggest that sex is still important to women who are depressed, but they also show that some antidepressants and the depression itself can interfere with sexual enjoyment. Are you having any problems?"

- When a patient has a chronic illness (eg, arthritis, multiple sclerosis, or diabetes mellitus), ask her: "Multiple sclerosis can sometimes interfere with a woman's sex life. Are you having any problems?"

- Before a potentially damaging surgery (eg, radical hysterectomy for cancer), explain to the patient: "The obvious need is to focus the surgery to remove the cancer entirely. The nerves and blood vessels that allow for sexual sensations and lubrication may be temporarily and occasionally permanently damaged. If sexual problems persist, they can be addressed. Do you have concerns now?"

- Before a bilateral elective oophorectomy for benign disease, explain to the patient: "Good evidence exists that women who choose to have both ovaries removed around the time of menopause when they need a hysterectomy do not develop subsequent sexual problems. Do you have concerns now?"

(continued)

Box 6. Establishing a Dialogue *(continued)*

- Before bilateral oophorectomy in younger women, explain to the patient: "Good evidence exists that women who choose to have both ovaries removed around menopause when they need a hysterectomy do not develop subsequent sexual problems. When women have to receive the same surgery when they are younger, and maybe feel they have no choice, especially if their family is not complete, they may sense changes in their sexuality. These can be addressed. Do you have concerns now?"

Diagnosis

Medical History

The patient's history is the crucial part of the assessment. The duration of the dysfunction and how it has evolved over time is clarified. Life-long problems are particularly difficult to evaluate and manage and concomitant in-depth psychologic assessment may be needed. The repercussions on the rest of the woman's sexual response and on that of her partner are detailed along with repercussions on their emotional intimacy. The context of her life when the dysfunction began is needed and should address psychologic, biologic, and relationship factors. The patient's medical history is recorded and should include medications and any substances of abuse. Past sexual experiences and relationships are explored, including any possible changes in orientation. Nonsexual and any sexual aspects of the woman's childhood and adolescence may be needed, particularly if her dysfunction is life-long. The most accurate information can be obtained if the couple is seen both together and individually. Clarifying confidentiality and expressing sensitivity and a nonjudgmental approach facilitates the gathering of information needed to establish not only a diagnosis but also the etiology of the condition and likely course of therapy.

The fundamental distinction between dysfunctions that are situational and those that are global or generalized is clinically relevant. Therefore, it is important to inquire about sexual response with masturbation, with viewing or reading erotica, and with being with persons other than the regular partner, even if this does not involve physical sexual interaction. These questions are asked only during the individual interviews. When the woman's sexual response alone is healthy but problematic with partnered sexual activity, she can be assured that her sexual response is intact. Her assessment will involve the interpersonal context, her thoughts and emotions during sexual encounters, her comfort with or fear of intimacy and vulnerability, and the details of the sexual context and stimuli.

Evaluation

FEMALE SEXUAL INTEREST/AROUSAL DISORDER

The woman's receptivity to the idea or request for sexual activity or any initiation by her is evaluated along with her ability to become aroused and to trigger desire to continue. Box 7 outlines the areas of inquiry.

Box 7. Women's Receptivity to Sexual Activity

- Sexual Motivation
  What causes her to instigate or accept sexual activity (eg, wanting or feeling emotional closeness, wish to experience sexual arousal, excitement with or without orgasm, wish to satisfy sexual desire/need, to show love/commitment, to feel attractive, to cause her partner to feel attractive, to feel normal, to relax, to keep a relationship, to avoid tension about sexual infrequency, or any other reasons)?

- Ability to Trigger Desire
  When she begins the sexual encounter without a sense of sexual desire can she become aroused? Once she is aroused and enjoying it, can she develop desire for sex for its own sake and other reasons she had initially?

  (continued)

Box 7. Women's Receptivity to Sexual Activity
(continued)

- Mental Sexual Arousal or Excitement
  What are the sources of the mental sexual arousal or excitement (eg, reading, hearing erotic or romantic talking, movies, stimulating her partner, receiving physical sexual stimulation, or deliberate recall of past sex or fantasy)?

- Awareness of Genital Response
  How does genital response manifest (eg, genital tingling, throbbing, sense of wanting genital touch or stimulation, or wetness)?

- Sensations From Genital Stimulation
  Does she have sensations from different forms of genital stimulation (eg, manual [her or her partner's fingers], oral stimulation, the use of vibrator, the use of dildo, or penile vulval stimulation)?

- Sensations From Penetrative Sex
  Does she have sensations from penetrative sex (eg, with entry, prolonged movements of intercourse or other penetration, continued movements after male partner's ejaculation, or combined manual and penetrative stimulation)?

- Thoughts During a Sexual Encounter
  What does she think about during a sexual encounter (eg, she gets distracted, she has worries about the outcome [eg, pain, privacy concerns, birth control or fertility concerns, or thoughts of being used or not appreciated])?

- Emotions During a Sexual Encounter
  What does she feel during a sexual encounter (eg, anxiety, shame, inadequacy, sadness, embarrassment, or guilt)?

FEMALE ORGASMIC DISORDER

When evaluating orgasmic disorder, the following unsatisfactory aspects should be determined:

- Is orgasm absent or extremely rare?
- Is orgasm very delayed?
- Is intensity of orgasm reduced?
- Are there also concerns with arousal?

For orgasm difficulties, it is important to check if this is truly generalized, ie, the difficulty persists with self-stimulation, partner's manual and oral stimulation, intercourse or other penetrative sex, or vibrator use, if she has tried this. Disorder is not diagnosed if some type of stimulation allows satisfactory orgasm.

GENITOPELVIC PAIN/PENETRATION DISORDER

When assessing genitopelvic pain/penetration disorder (formerly known as dyspareunia or vaginismus), it is important to inquire if vaginal entry is possible at all, ie, with finger, penis, dildo, speculum, or tampon. Women are hesitant to admit that penile–vaginal intercourse, ie, penetrative sex, has never been possible, and this possibility must be raised. Also, it must be established whether or not she is sexually aroused as the attempt begins and progresses.

When fear prevents penile or dildo contact with the introitus, and entry has not occurred, the physician should initially inquire what attempts at vaginal entry have been made (eg, the partner's finger, tampon, a physician's finger, or speculum), how complete these have been, and what emotions were present during these experiences. If fear is present, the patient should be asked to clarify exactly of what she is fearful. Any previous attempted internal examination should be discussed. The physician should confirm whether the woman wants to address this problem now and whether other major stressors are currently present in her life. Dealing with phobic avoidance of vaginal entry can be immensely stressful. Presence of the following symptoms, which suggest provoked vestibulodynia, should be clearly established:

- Vulval burning with partner ejaculation onto introitus
- Dysuria after attempt at vaginal entry

- Vulval discomfort for minutes or hours after penetration attempt

Although fear and phobic avoidance constitute the usual etiology, introital anatomical abnormalities or erectile dysfunction in a male partner or a lack of sexual skills or information are possible.

When partial or full vaginal entry is possible but painful, the physician should inquire exactly when the pain is experienced, as per following situations:

- With partial entry of penis or dildo
- With attempted full entry of penile head or dildo
- With deep thrusting
- With penile or dildo movement
- With a male partner's ejaculation
- With woman's subsequent urination
- For hours or minutes after intercourse or penetration attempts

Physical Examination

Physical examination is crucial in women with some sexual disorders. Genital examination may show scant or absent pubic hair clinically associated with a history of past excessive stress or less often with past Sheehan syndrome. Chronic dyspareunia requires a careful genital examination, especially of the introitus because in most cases of dyspareunia, the pain is introital. Careful detailed inspection for vulval atrophy or dystrophy or posterior fourchette scars of past splitting is facilitated by allowing the woman to see the areas of examination using a mirror. Also, she may wish to observe the testing for allodynia of provoked vestibulodynia around the hymenal edge with a cotton-tipped swab. If her anxiety is marked, she may prefer to do the cotton-tipped swab test herself with physician guidance. Resting vaginal tone can be approximately assessed by the examining finger, and voluntary muscle contraction and relaxation also can be assessed. Tenderness, often focal from pressing on the deep levator ani ring, can be checked along with pain and discomfort from palpating the uterus and adnexa. Fixed retroversion can be detected, along with any nodularity suggestive of endometriosis. Bladder and urethral sensitivity should be assessed by palpating the anterior vaginal wall.

The results of a detailed examination for lifelong orgasmic disorder usually are normal. Nevertheless, it is reassuring to the woman to know that her physical examination results are normal. In cases of acquired orgasmic disorder, especially in the presence of neurologic disease, the examination is important and requires additional neurologic testing. Cold sensation from the clitoris can usefully be detected using cold lubricant gel. This modality of sensory testing is clinically more relevant to orgasm potential than the use of touch. The motor aspect of the orgasm reflex, ie, S2–S4 pudendal nerves, can be checked by asking the woman to voluntarily contract the muscles around the vagina or the anus. The vulvar area should be examined for vulvar dystrophy: loss of orgasm may be associated with lichen sclerosis.

The pelvic examination for women with hypoactive sexual desire disorder has limited usefulness. A general physical examination for acquired loss of desire is reasonable although clues to any systemic illness usually would have been found when the medical history was obtained.

Laboratory Tests

Currently available laboratory investigations are of limited value. Estrogen status usually is detected by medical history and examination, although on occasion estradiol level assessments are needed. Follicle-stimulating hormone testing around perimenopause is of limited value given the marked fluctuations in levels; measurement of anti-Müllerian hormone levels might be indicated. Measurement of testosterone levels is useful only to investigate signs of hirsutism or clitoromegaly. Recent research confirms that even with access to mass spectrometry assays neither serum levels of testosterone nor of total androgen metabolites are associated with sexual dysfunction (98). When infertility or oligomenorrhea are present, the prolactin level is measured to account for low desire. When relevant symptoms or signs are present, the level of thyroid-stimulating hormone is measured. Vaginal, cervical, and vulval specimens for culture may be indicated in women with chronic dyspareunia. Objective measurement of vaginal congestion during arousal with plethysmograph is not routinely available in most clinics. Other pelvic imaging techniques are currently investigational as is any brain imaging during exposure to sexual stimuli.

Coexisting Factors

MEDICATIONS

The most common medications associated with sexual dysfunction are the SSRIs. Delay or absence of orgasm with reduced sexual desire occurs in up to 70% of women who take SSRIs. The clinical observation is that antidepressants that activate dopaminergic, noradrenergic (central), and 5HT1A and 5HT2C receptors may augment sexual response, whereas those that activate other 5HT receptors, prolactin, and GABA reduce sexual response. Therefore, those medications that are least likely to interfere include the following:

- Serotonergic agents sparing 5HT2 receptor, eg, mirtazapine
- Agents with central noradrenergic action, eg, mirtazapine, bupropion, venlafaxine, and duloxetine
- Agents with dopaminergic action, eg, bupropion and venlafaxine
- Agents that are 5HT1A agonists, eg, buspirone

The sexual benefits of adequately treating depression far outweigh the potential negative sexual adverse effects of the medications. A serotonin–norepinephrine reuptake inhibitor, duloxetine, may lessen sexual function also but to a smaller extent than an SSRI. Agomelatine, available in Europe, is an agonist of melatonin receptors MT1 and MT2 and antagonist of 5HT2C. It has minimal sexual effects comparable with placebo and significantly less than paroxetine or venlafaxine.

Opinion varies as to whether epilepsy per se or the use of anticonvulsants lessens sexual desire. Many women can take anticonvulsants for diseases other than epilepsy without sexual adverse effects. Antipsychotics can frequently delay orgasm.

Narcotics typically reduce sexual desire and motivation. A sub-group of women who take oral contraceptives report low sexual desire, but recent studies do not support the connection between low desire and dysfunction and oral contraceptives. Limited research suggests raloxifene and tamoxifen are not associated with sexual adverse effects. Dyspareunia from aromatase inhibitors is common. Phytoestrogens may exacerbate vaginal dryness and dyspareunia.

MEDICAL CONDITIONS

Women's sexual dysfunctions are robustly linked to depression. Low desire is almost universal in women who have major depression, but arousal, lubrication, and orgasm also may be impaired. Depression is the major factor that influences sexual function in women with chronic illness, including end-stage renal disease, multiple sclerosis, or diabetes and those after bone marrow transplantation (135). Anxiety disorders are associated with increased prevalence of sexual dysfunction, especially provoked vestibulodynia (136). An association is possible between women with obsessive–compulsive disorder and orgasmic disorder and past sexual abuse. Chronic conditions that affect energy, well-being, and self-image may indirectly affect sexual desire and response, such as cardiac or renal failure, arthritis, and cancer (137). Neurologic conditions, including multiple sclerosis, spinal cord injury, cerebrovascular disease or trauma, and Parkinson disease, frequently limit sexuality in multiple ways (137). Conditions that interfere with the hormonal milieu can interfere with sex response and include Addison disease, hypopituitary states, nonelective bilateral salpingo-oophorectomy, hyperprolactinemia, hypothyroid and hyperthyroid states, metabolic syndrome, and the hormonal disruption from iatrogenic menopause and aromatase inhibition for breast cancer.

PARTNER SEXUAL DYSFUNCTION

Any partner dysfunction can reduce women's sexual response. Commonly, this includes erectile dysfunction, premature ejaculation in male partners, and desire or orgasm difficulty in female partners.

PSYCHOLOGIC FACTORS

Psychologic factors commonly affect sexual response (Box 8). As explained previously, these factors continuously modulate sexual motivation and arousal experienced from sexual stimuli. They influence the woman's motivation to find or attend to those sexual stimuli, thus compounding any negative effects from biologic factors.

SEXUAL ABUSE

Many researchers report a relationship between childhood sexual abuse and female sexual dysfunction. However, past studies have been limited not only by small numbers but also by the omission of comparison groups. Lack of a comparison group is relevant

---

Box 8. Psychologic Factors

- Depression
- Anxiety
- Effects of medications
- Fatigue—sleep deprivation, poor timing, poor health, or shift work
- Stress—work-, family-, or financial-related
- Interpersonal issues
- Lack of useful stimuli or environment
- Limited sexual communication
- Past experiences—past negative or abusive sexual experiences
- Negative self-image—premature menopause, disfiguring surgery, or incontinence
- Difficulty remaining focused
- Expectation of a negative outcome—partner sexual dysfunction, pain, lack of emotional closeness, or absence of orgasm

because of the high percentage of women who, during routine gynecologic care, report sexual problems (138). Although studies of college students typically report few differences in sexual function between abused and nonabused students, community studies and especially clinical studies tend to show an increased incidence of sexual dysfunction in abused women compared with controls. Low desire, difficulties with arousal and orgasm, feeling little sexual sensation, lack of sexual satisfaction, and sexual avoidance are all reported (139). Abuse that involved penetration or violence is specifically related to adult sexual dysfunction. One review reports problems with orgasm to be the most common concern that affects some 45% of women with childhood sexual abuse histories (140). Noted is the fact that a large number of women with childhood sexual abuse histories report satisfactory sexual lives, and research is needed to determine other factors that increase the risk of dysfunction. The study suggests the tendency to avoid interpersonal closeness and emotional involvement predicts orgasm difficulty (140).

Management

A detailed, sensitive, and respectful assessment will help establish a dialogue with the patient. It is difficult to clearly distinguish between assessment and management because the physician often provides information during the assessment that is therapeutic.

Psychotherapeutic methods (141) are the mainstay of management of the female sexual dysfunction (for a systematic review, see section "Resources"). Box 9 lists psychologic and biologic interventions that can be used in gynecologic offices.

Female Sexual Interest/Arousal Disorder

To manage a patient with sexual interest/arousal disorder, obstetrician–gynecologists can refer to the circular model of sexual response (Fig. 1) to discuss with one or preferably both partners which areas are problematic. Some problems may be addressed by the obstetrician–gynecologist and others may necessitate referral. When lack of sufficient emotional intimacy is identified, the

Box 9. Psychologic and Biologic Interventions

- Giving nonjudgmental and respectful information about sexual function and dysfunction

- Applying the model of women's responsive or triggered desire to the patient (and partner)

- Explain to both partners that nonpenetrative sex is normal, that many women need nonphysical, physical nongenital, and genital nonpenetrative stimulation, and any of these may be more rewarding than vaginal penetration

- Screening for depression and sexual adverse effects of antidepressants—consider changing to mirtazapine, venlafaxine, duloxetine, or bupropion or add bupropion to a selective serotonin reuptake inhibitor. Other measures are not evidence based, and interrupting the use of short-acting selective serotonin reuptake inhibitors for the sake of a sexual encounter risks return of depressive symptoms or withdrawal symptoms and possible future adherence

- Screening for other medication-associated female sexual dysfunction and advising alternative medications (eg, for β-blockers, consider changing to an alternative drug as guided by the clinical situation)

- Addressing fatigue

- Prescribing estrogen locally or systemically

- Treating hyperprolactinemia, hypothyroidism, or hyperthyroidism

- Addressing insecurity regarding birth control or sexually transmitted disease

- Addressing and managing fear of urinary incontinence during sex

(continued)

Box 9. Psychologic and Biologic Interventions
(continued)

- Explaining that desire discrepancy is normal (ie, most couples have to negotiate an endeavor to make sexual encounters as rewarding as possible— the partner with lower sexual need can still participate in somewhat more encounters than the preferred frequency with genuine enjoyment [as opposed to simple participation] and the partner with the higher sexual need can accept that sexual encounters will be less frequent than is desired; no standard or normal frequency for sexual encounters exists)

"normality" of low interest to be sexual can be clarified; referral for couple counseling may be indicated. When the lack of sexual context and stimuli are contributing factors, simply emphasizing this need usually is sufficient, but referral to sex therapists may be appropriate. Studies of placebo response are enlightening. In the female trials of tadalafil (phosphodiesterase inhibitor approved for erectile dysfunction), a statistically significant positive response was reported by one third of placebo recipients, similar to that of patients who received active drugs. A positive response was found to be linked to changes in sexual behavior of the couple during the trial rather than to age, severity of symptoms, or duration (142).

Figure 4 shows the main modalities of treatment, namely cognitive behavioral therapy, sex therapy, and psychoeducation. New to Western medicine is the addition of mindfulness, which has already shown promise in therapy of sexual dysfunction in medically healthy women (143) and in those with pelvic cancer (144) and with provoked vestibulodynia (145, 146). Mindfulness is an Eastern practice with roots in Buddhist meditation, which focuses on present moment, nonjudgmental awareness. Its practice allows attention to sexual sensations rather than to distractions. Functional brain imaging before and after mindfulness

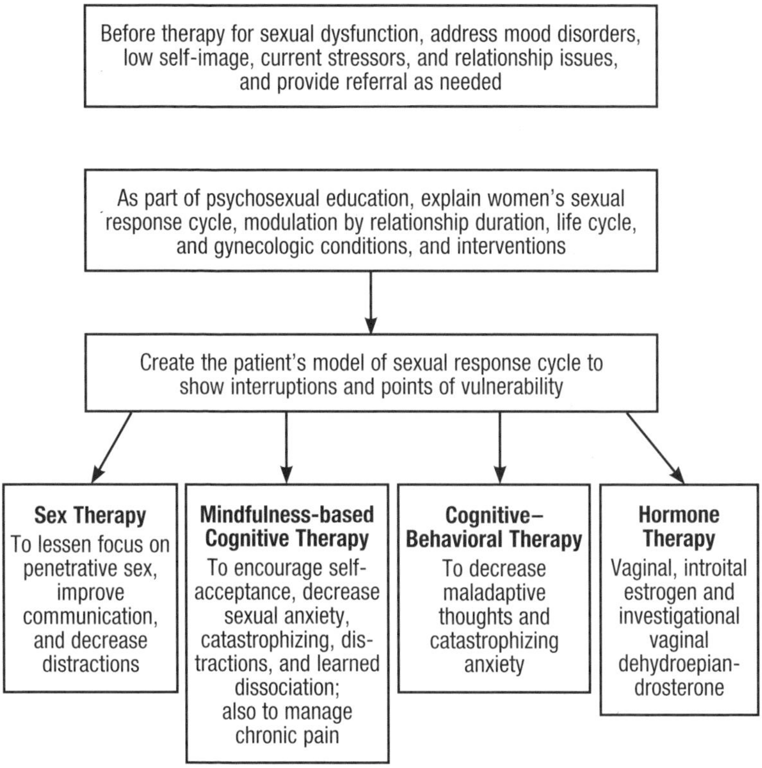

Fig. 4. Main modalities of treatment of women's sexual dysfunction. Comorbidity of difficulties with desire, arousal, and orgasm with or without pain is typical.

training supports the clinical finding that such training decreases self-referencing of sensations and emotions, including pain and anxiety (147–149). Resources in the community and through the Internet for mindfulness practice can be given to patients (see section "Resources").

Standard sex therapy can be explained and referral made to a sex therapist, if needed. Sensate focus exercises can be outlined by the obstetrician–gynecologist, possibly to accompany mindfulness practice. Sensate focus exercises involve each partner taking turns giving and receiving sensual, and later on, sexual touches, caresses, and kisses. Initially, genital areas and breasts are off-limits. The idea of any goal or expectation is put aside. Usually, each session lasts 15–20 minutes and two or preferably three sessions should occur each week for 3–6 weeks. The couple together with the clinician decides as to when breasts and genital areas are included. Ultimately, the act of intercourse (vaginal penetration with dildo) may be included. For some women with chronic disease or cancer, intercourse may not be possible at all, and the couple should be encouraged to include more erotic and various nonpenetrative activities.

Cognitive–behavioral therapy may be recommended by the gynecologist. This can assist the woman to recognize her negative and often catastrophic self-view imposed by illness, including gynecologic conditions or infertility. Some women view themselves as sexually substandard, feeling that they do not "deserve" reasonable treatment in a relationship, and thus will even remain in abusive relationships. Other exaggerated or catastrophic thoughts amenable to cognitive therapy include "sex is only for well women," "I am no longer fertile; I am no longer sexually attractive," and "if intercourse is impossible, then no one will want me." Empiric support for efforts to address cognitions and emotions during sex is increasing (150, 151), which can benefit physical and subjective arousal (150).

Recently, an adapted form of cognitive–behavioral therapy blended with mindfulness was defined—the treatment is called *mindfulness-based cognitive therapy*. Regular mindfulness practice is an integral component. Also, the skill of detecting maladaptive thoughts is learned, but with mere observation of their presence and an acknowledgment that they are just mental events and by no means are they necessarily the truth. Mindfulness-based cognitive therapy is used to treat anxiety disorder and depression and to prevent recurrent depression and has been adapted to treat arousal and desire disorders and chronic pain of provoked vestibulodynia (75, 146, 152, 153).

Data are limited regarding the long-term effects of psychologic treatments for women's sexual dysfunction. A systematic review and a meta-analysis of controlled clinical trials for female and male sexual dysfunction have been published (154). Fifteen studies of women were identified plus two studies that reviewed dysfunction in males and females. However, for women, most studies involved sexual pain; only four studies involved hypoactive desire and three, orgasmic disorder. Although involving both partners in therapy generally is recommended, nine studies involved only the patient. Most research involved small group therapy—cognitive–behavioral therapy, sex therapy, or both. The overall conclusion was that psychosocial interventions for sexual dysfunctions were efficacious. The meta-analysis included fourteen studies of female patients who receive interventions compared with those who were put on a waitlist. A clear evidence of benefit was documented for symptom severity and sexual satisfaction in women with orgasmic dysfunction and women with low desire. For women with sexual dysfunction after breast cancer, a systematic review suggests that the most effective interventions are couple-based psychoeducational interventions that include an element of sexual therapy (155).

For many decades, women's age-related reduction in androgen activity plus possible iatrogenic loss of ovarian androgens has been assumed to contribute to reduced desire and arousal, leading to an off-label prescription of testosterone. The latter has markedly increased in recent years but is not evidence-based. Using accurate serum assays, neither total androgen activity nor levels of testosterone are decreased in women in whom hypoactive sexual desire disorder is diagnosed (98) and in those with comorbid arousal disorder (152). Support is limited for the use of investigational systemic testosterone supplementation in estrogen-replete postmenopausal women who can have two to three satisfying sexual events per month; importantly, such women do not fulfill a diagnosis of sexual interest/arousal disorder (53). No discriminatory value for serum testosterone or serum androgen metabolites exists below which testosterone might usefully be supplemented to improve desire (45). Testosterone therapy is not recommended for general use by the Endocrine Society or by the International Society for Sexual Medicine (45, 156). Despite the identified decrease in DHEA with age, a review indicates that systemic DHEA therapy does not benefit women with female sexual dysfunction (105). Guidelines from the 2010 International Consensus on Sexual Medicine state that any decision to use testosterone therapy must be individualized (156). However, since then, the two negative trials of testosterone gel (LibiGel) have been reported (114). Women in the trial were able to have two to three satisfying sexual events per

month at baseline. Thus, the previously reported benefit from
transdermal systemic testosterone therapy to such women was
not confirmed. The lack of publication of trials with negative
results, over and beyond an abstract form, means that many clinicians are unaware of the conflicting evidence on testosterone
therapy. If obstetrician–gynecologists prescribe testosterone,
these conflicting data on any benefit, the absence of "disorder"
as currently understood in the recruited women, its investigational nature, and the lack of long-term safety data must be
explained to the patient along with need for careful follow-up.
The concerns regarding co-administered long-term systemic
estrogen also must be disclosed. No formulations designed for
women are available.

Tibolone, an agent with estrogenic, progestogenic, and
androgenic action was shown repeatedly to increase desire and
response scores in sexually functional women recruited for nonsexual reasons for postmenopausal therapy. However, an RCT of
sexually dysfunctional women showed benefit only comparable
with that afforded by transdermal estradiol and norethisterone
acetate (121).

Nonhormonal medications have been investigated but the
trials have been discontinued. Included were flibanserin (5HTA
agonist, 5HT2A antagonist, and weak D4 agonist), tadalafil, and
sildenafil (phosphodiesterase type-5 inhibitors). Trials of bremelanotide (an agonist at MT1, MT3, and MT4 receptors) were
discontinued because of increases in blood pressure. A different
pharmaceutical company is again conducting a clinical trial of
the drug with intranasal or subcutaneous delivery. Concerns of
risk remain because of the involvement of melatonin in multiple
systems. Investigational use of intravaginal DHEA, 13 mg nightly,
may restore atrophy-associated loss of genital sexual sensitivity
and promote arousal and orgasm (131) (see the section "Vulvovaginal Atrophy") thereby increasing sexual interest.

Orgasmic Disorder

Most women referred to gynecologists who report orgasmic
difficulty also experience only low levels of arousal. For those
women who are able to be highly aroused, but distressed that

they cannot release that arousal, the following management strategies can be considered:

- Management of psychologic factors

  —Fear of losing control—encouragement to self-stimulate may be helpful.

  —Lack of trust of others, including their partners—a referral to psychologist should be considered.

  —Fear of closeness because of a fear of loss should the relationship end—the patient should be referred to a sex therapist or psychologist.

- Management of biologic factors

  —Autonomic nerve damage—increased stimulation, especially vibrostimulation should be considered.

  —Selective serotonin reuptake inhibitor-associated female orgasmic disorder—bupropion (limited evidence of benefit; 79), or sildenafil (one study with very strict entry criteria suggested benefit; 157) may be added, or it may be possible to replace an SSRI with an antidepressant with fewer sex-related adverse affects.

For all these situations, increasing the number and intensity of stimuli, such as mental imagery and fantasy, visual, tactile, auditory, and written, may be helpful—simultaneously, if necessary. Stimulation with a vibrator or with a clitoral therapy device may benefit women with or without nerve damage. The clitoral therapy device creates a vacuum over the superficial parts of the clitoris, which increases their engorgement from sexual stimulation. The device has not been studied in comparison with vibrators that appear clinically to be superior in benefit and acceptability, but one uncontrolled pilot study found benefit in women after radiation therapy for cervical cancer (158). Of note is the extensive clitoral tissue deep to the labia and superficial muscles that is effectively sexually stimulated by hand or by partner's body; the superficial shaft and head alone are engorged by creating vacuum, and clinical experience is that this is rarely helpful. However, the device has been approved by the U.S. Food and Drug Administration.

Cognitive–behavioral therapy has been found across studies to be highly effective as a short-term therapy for women with life-long female orgasmic disorder (159). Three RCTs are published (160–162). Two specific forms of cognitive–behavioral therapy to consider as first-line treatments are guided or directed self-stimulation and coital alignment technique. Directed self-stimulation is used most frequently and involves education and information followed by body awareness exercises designed to enhance women's awareness of their genitals and to challenge any negative or distorted thoughts that might emerge. A useful book is *Becoming Orgasmic* by Julia Heiman (see the section "Resources"). The exercises progressively increase in intensity, including using a hand-held mirror to enhance sensory experience until the woman learns to reach orgasm on her own. She is then taught how to transfer this new knowledge to a partner. Success rates for directed self-stimulation are high (80–90%), but the success rate for secondary female orgasmic disorder is lower (10–75%) (163). Coital alignment technique is a behavioral technique, which allows increased pubis-to-pubis contact between partners during intercourse. It may be possible to obtain only after a male partner's ejaculation and partial detumescence. One study that directly compared coital alignment technique with directed self-stimulation for women with secondary female orgasmic disorder found that coital alignment technique produced a significantly better response (164).

Mindfulness, as mentioned previously, involves learning to be present in the moment and not react to potentially negative feelings or thoughts and simply to observe them and return to the sexual sensations. Although scientific study of the benefits is only just beginning, clinical experience supports the use of this meditative skill for female orgasmic disorder.

Dyspareunia

At least three components are involved in the management of chronic dyspareunia:

1. Definitive treatment for the underlying gynecologic condition (or the underlying lack of arousal)

2. Explanation of the effects of chronic dyspareunia on the woman's sexual response cycle—the sexual infrequency

that typically accompanies chronic dyspareunia often leads to guilt and anxiety about the relationship, which in turn are distracting during sexual stimulation and preclude pleasure, arousal, or orgasm.

3. Explanation of the need to remove any painful aspect of sexual experiences, ie, to support the need, at least, temporarily for only nonpenetrative sex—removing the painful component can be endorsed by the gynecologist who can explain that rewarding sexual experiences can allow sexual motivation to return. Viewing sex as something the patient wants to do as opposed to it being "just for the sake of her partner" is an important component of her recovery.

VULVOVAGINAL ATROPHY

First-line therapy is local administration of estrogen in the form of a vaginal tablet or cream or a silastic ring (165). Smaller doses of these formulations are being investigated (eg, 10-microgram rather than 100-microgram estradiol cream) or have already been approved (eg, 10-microgram rather than 100-microgram estradiol cream or 0.03-mg rather than 0.2-mg estriol vaginal pessaries). The estrogen ring that releases 7.5 micrograms daily leads to serum levels of 8 pg/mL compared with 4.6 pg/mL from the 10-microgram estradiol tablet. Conjugated equine estrogen cream is approved for dyspareunia at doses ranging from 0.3 mg to 1.25 mg and the frequency ranging from daily to weekly. Serum levels may slightly exceed the normal postmenopausal range. A hyaluronic acid vaginal gel has been shown to improve symptoms in 85% of women, comparable with women who received vaginal estriol. However, only the latter agent decreased the pH (166). Symptoms from vulvovaginal atrophy may remit spontaneously within 1 year; risk factors for more severe symptoms are diabetes, younger age, and low body mass index (167). The traditional notion that maintaining sexual activity will prevent symptomatic vulvovaginal atrophy has been refuted (3). Subjective symptoms and objective signs of vulvovaginal atrophy correlate poorly (168). Psychologic factors rather than estrogen levels were shown to moderate symptoms when vulvovaginal atrophy is present (89).

Also, postmenopausal vulvovaginal atrophy-associated dyspareunia may be accompanied by provoked vestibulodynia (169).

A study of vaginal DHEA, 6.5–13 mg nightly (131) or another study of adding 0.5 mg 2%-testosterone to biweekly 0.625 mg conjugated equine estrogen cream (133) suggests a sexual benefit in addition to coital comfort. Systemic therapy is an alternative option in some recently menopausal women but a marked caution exists concerning long-term systemic estrogen therapy as a result of just one large and not particularly clinically relevant study. The Women's Health Initiative (WHI) trial did not focus on women with sexual and vasomotor symptoms associated with menopause who subsequently began systemic estrogen (ie, at a time when asymptomatic coronary artery disease would be less prevalent) (170). Reviewers of observational and randomized trials to date conclude that young symptomatic menopausal women who use estrogen therapy for long periods have less mortality and coronary heart disease than comparable women without such therapy. Nevertheless, a reduced incidence of breast cancer that has followed reduced prescriptions of postmenopausal HT subsequent to the WHI trial adds to the need for caution.

Provoked Vestibulodynia

Provoked vestibulodynia affects women of all ages and is believed to be the most common form of chronic premenopausal dyspareunia; the latter affects some 12–21% of women. Diagnostic criteria of provoked vestibulodynia include severe pain on vestibular touch, marked tenderness to cotton swab palpation of the vulvar vestibule, and physical findings within normal limits. The provoking stimulus is typically the attempted entry and movement of penis or dildo but also can be a speculum, tampon, or menstrual cup insertion, or even tight clothing seams. Subsequent sexual dysfunction is common (171). Multiple etiologic factors for provoked vestibulodynia have been considered and range from genetic predisposition, genital infections, "microtrauma" to the vulva, aberrant immune reactions to *Candida albicans*, to possibly unknown irritants to the vestibule leading to altered sensitivity of the dorsal horn cells of the spinal cord, which receive the increased afferent (incoming) nociceptive (painful) signals. Comorbidity with other pain syndromes is frequently documented, most notably with irritable bowel syndrome and fibromyalgia. Hyperalgesia and decreased pain thresholds in nongenital parts of the body have been demonstrated in women with provoked vestibulodynia who generally report more bodily pain compared with a normal population. Although knowledge of chronic pain physiology is limited, recent research into the changes that reflect neuroplasticity inherent in the brain and spinal cord sheds some light on such comorbidity and pain hypersensitivity. Current understanding of provoked vestibulodynia supports the possibility that provoked vestibulodynia reflects stress-induced dysregulation of the CNS (75) as suggested for other pain disorders (172–174). Depression and anxiety disorders commonly precede provoked vestibulodynia and also may occur subsequently to the onset of pain (136). Reviews of provoked vestibulodynia and the four published randomized controlled trials confirm the clinical impression that medical modalities of treatment are largely unsatisfactory (175, 176). Although results of limited outcome studies of surgical management (vestibulectomy) appear promising, exclusion criteria are extensive (eg, depression, unwillingness to also have sexual counseling or pelvic muscle physiotherapy, lifelong symptoms, and involvement of the areas adjacent to the urethra). Also, the allodynia may improve after surgery but intercourse may not be resumed (177). Pelvic muscle physiotherapy and biofeedback are useful adjuncts, but the increased muscle tone may not only be reflexive because of introital tenderness but also be part of the pain syndrome and require measures to address the underlying stress. Emerging research of adapting two psychologic therapies, namely cognitive–behavioral therapy and mindfulness (ie, mindfulness-based cognitive therapy), suggests improvements in pain and sexual function (146, 152, 153). Because of its potential compounding effects on pain intensity, sexual dysfunction needs to be addressed along with pain management (75). The appeal of such therapy, in contrast to local medical or surgical treatment, is the potential benefit to frequently comorbid pain syndromes, including irritable bowel syndrome and fibromyalgia. The number of concomitant pain syndromes has been linked to poor provoked vestibulodynia treatment outcomes (178). Also, mindfulness-based cognitive therapy is of benefit in women with frequently occurring comorbid depression and anxiety disorders and the frequently comorbid sexual interest/arousal disorder.

Numerous functional MRI studies have delineated a constellation of brain regions activated during pain. Imaging of individuals with a chronic pain syndrome who receive a deliberate invoking of that pain show brain activity that is enhanced and different from when they (or participants in control groups) receive a different acute painful stimulus (179). Functional MRI research in women with provoked vestibulodynia demonstrated similar pain augmentation when the painful stimulus was applied to a site remote from the vulva, such as the thumb, which suggests changes within the CNS in provoked vestibulodynia (180). These findings are in keeping with hyperalgesia and decreased pain thresholds in nongenital parts of the body in women with provoked vestibulodynia (181).

Functional brain imaging of pain processes suggests that mindfulness training may lead to altered pain processing when a painful stimulus is given even when individuals who practice it are not formally meditating (182, 183). A review found that imaging data to date supported the clinical experience that mindfulness training enables an individual to accept an effective state (including pain) as an object of attention and that this was related to an enhanced ability to engage frontal cortical structures to diminish amygdala activation (184).

An interdisciplinary approach and a focus on mind skills to ameliorate the chronic pain of provoked vestibulodynia are showing promise (146, 152, 153). The skills of cognitive–behavioral therapy, mindfulness, and, more recently, mindfulness-based cognitive therapy can be taught in a small group format of typically six to eight women with two facilitators.

CASE NO. 1. A 30-year-old woman had a consultation for sexual difficulties. She reported a 4-year unconsummated marriage. The patient had a long-term fear of pain from vaginal entry and had never attempted to use a tampon. She reported pain with multiple attempts to allow penile entry, most of which occurred in the first year of marriage.

Before marriage, the partners practiced nonpenetrative sex with arousal and orgasms for both partners. Little nonpenetrative sex had occurred in the past 3 years. The patient had lost motivation for any type of sexual interaction with her husband and had never self-stimulated. Her husband was supportive, understanding, and concerned that he might cause her pain. He was willing to wait until her condition is treated. This patient also has irritable bowel syndrome. Her primary care provider and a fertility specialist had been unable to perform a pelvic examination because of the patient's fear of vaginal penetration.

Initial management included counseling. The couple was advised to discontinue any attempts at vaginal penetration, and the patient was encouraged to spend 5–10 minutes each day for nonsexual self-touch. Initially, this would involve the labia majora and later when felt ready, the labia majora. Later, she was encouraged to separate the labia majora gently but sufficiently to expose the introitus and envision this practice as a means to allow the physician to inspect the vulva, including the introitus.

When seen 3 weeks later, the patient was ready for a partial gynecologic examination. With the examination table adjusted so she was less vulnerable than lying flat and also able to see herself in a hand-held mirror, she was encouraged to use abdominal breathing to relax before being asked to open the labia as she had practiced. She watched in the mirror as her normal anatomy was pointed out by the physician. She was unable to perform a voluntary Kegel tightening of the pelvic floor muscles or a reverse Kegel maneuver so that her perineum could descend. Nevertheless, she was able to see the introitus open when she coughed, and with the aid of coughing could insert her own finger through the introitus into the vagina. She permitted the physician to perform a single digit examination, which confirmed markedly heightened tone of the pelvic floor. The result of the cotton-swab test for allodynia of provoked vestibulodynia was positive; all points on the introital rim were scored at 10 points out of 10 in pain intensity.

The comorbid conditions of provoked vestibulodynia and the condition previously called vaginismus were explained. Home practice of insertion of her own finger was encouraged. The patient was referred to a small group program that consisted of eight weekly 2.5-hour sessions that focused on psychologic approaches to chronic pain, especially mindfulness-based cognitive therapy. Aided by treatment manuals and education during the sessions, the women learned some of the pathophysiology of provoked vestibulodynia, mechanisms of chronic pain, and the likely role of stress in provoked vestibulodynia. For the next few weeks, the women were encouraged to practice nonpenetrative sex. For women who still reported painful intercourse, this was a way to break the cycle of expected and experienced pain. This patient could resume nonpenetrative sex while knowing that no attempt at penetration would occur. A major part of the program was devoted to mindfulness practice. Information also was given regarding the potential consequences of provoked vestibulodynia on sexual desire, motivation, and response.

At a 6-month follow-up visit, the patient reported a pregnancy (5 weeks of gestation). The couple has resumed nonpenetrative sex. The patient has used a series of vaginal inserts to assist the muscle accommodation reflex and continued with her daily mindfulness practice. She had been able to undergo a pelvic examination. The couple then used a syringe for insemination. On examination, a decreased "vaginistic" muscle response was reported—allodynia was still present, rated as a score of 4 out of 10. At a 12-month follow-up visit, the pregnancy was progressing well. Neither partner had wanted to advance to include intercourse in their sexual activity together, preferring to wait until after the pregnancy. Their questions concerning a delivery in women with provoked vestibulodynia were addressed. A vaginal delivery with an epidural anesthesia at full term occurred. One year later, intercourse had not been attempted, with neither partner voicing any distress. Nonpenetrative sex continued.

This case illustrates the overlap of vaginismus and provoked vestibulodynia in keeping with the new *DSM-5* classification of sexual pain, ie, genitopelvic penetration disorder. Also, it illustrates that "vaginismus" typically is an entity that involves both partners being hesitant about penetrative sex.

CASE NO. 2. A 38-year-old woman was seen by your colleague in your office. She explained that currently, she was single but had two previous 3-year relationships with female partners and six short relationships with male partners. Burning introital pain that was consistent throughout intercourse and penetration and the subsequent 30–60 minutes has been present since her second relationship. The patient noted her first partner had a small penis, and no pain was present with intercourse in that 2-year relationship in her late adolescence.

Her sexual desire and motivation to be with her partner in the two most recent relationships remained high, and arousal is prompt and orgasms enjoyable. Self-stimulation continues, but she avoids inserting objects into the vagina. In her past two relationships, if her partner's fingers or a dildo was inserted vaginally, pain was consistently present especially with movement and would cause up to 2 hours of vulvodynia after sexual activity.

Medical history of this patient is significant for irritable bowel syndrome, temporomandibular joint pain, and panic attacks. Past treatment of the introital pain was unhelpful—the patient had felt dismissed once she explained her sexual orientation. She was prescribed a steroid ointment but noted no benefit. On the examination of the introital rim, this patient had allodynia rated at 8–9 points out of 10 points at all locations except for the 6 o'clock point, where the pain was significantly decreased. Pelvic muscle tone was increased. Although she was able to perform a Kegel contraction, she was unable to relax the pelvic floor. The patient was referred to the same small group program as the patient from Case No. 1. The sessions encouraged this patient to begin with nonpenetrative sex in her next relationship.

At a 6-month follow-up, the patient was in a new lesbian relationship. Her desire, arousal, and orgasm remained healthy. The couple included vaginal penetration in their sexual activity, and this was without pain. On examination, allodynia remained at a score of 3 to 4 out of 10.

This case was atypical in that the patient's sexual response remained healthy despite the chronic pain. Importantly, she was able to negotiate nonpenetrative sex with her partners when this was necessary. Subsequent to cognitive therapy for provoked vestibulodynia, often patients can be pain-free when sexually active with penetration because they have learned that their control and reward from sex can lessen or remove pain. However, when the mind is focused on pain intensity, as in the gynecologic examination with a cotton-tipped swab, allodynia is present to some degree despite reports of pain-free sex.

> **CASE NO. 3.** A 58-year-old woman reported introital pain since menopause at age 53 years. Various modalities had been tried with no benefit and varied adverse effects. Among the modalities tried were topical formulations of estrogen, which provided no improvement; a 3-month treatment with amitriptyline, which did not relieve the pain but caused sedation; and pelvic muscle physiotherapy, which confirmed and addressed heightened pelvic muscle tone but did not improve dyspareunia. The patient described her current level of sexual desire and arousal as low with rare orgasms. Although before menopause, she occasionally self-stimulated to orgasm, this also had stopped. The patient's husband insists on penetrative sex, refuses to acknowledge the patient's condition, and does not accompany her to the clinic. Fibromyalgia was diagnosed 5 years ago and temporomandibular jaw pain has been present for the past 2 years. No past diagnosis of mood disorders was reported; however, the patient feels that she had postpartum depression after two of her three pregnancies. On examination, signs of vulvovaginal atrophy were present. Allodynia also was present at a score of 10 out of 10 in all areas. Neither Kegel exercises nor reverse Kegel maneuvers were possible, and pelvic muscle tone was high.
>
> The dual diagnoses of provoked vestibulodynia and vulvovaginal atrophy were explained. Clinical experience favors topical estriol over estradiol for allodynia and postmenopausal provoked vestibulodynia. This was explained along with the need for a chronic pain approach. A twice-weekly vaginal application of 0.3 mg topical estriol along with local

nightly application at the introital rim was prescribed. The patient was shown how to place the cream accurately in the deep crease between the outer edge of the hymen and inner edge of the labia minora. In addition, the patient was referred to the same small group therapy program as the patients from Case No. 1 and Case No. 2. For this patient, the information and techniques learned in the program seemed logical but impossible to apply because of her husband's attitude.

At a 6-month follow-up visit, the patient explained that her husband had agreed to attend a two-session group therapy for male partners of women with provoked vestibulodynia that included mindfulness practice. As a result, the couple was able to experience nonpenetrative sex. On examination, the allodynia was still present at a score of 6 to 7 out of 10 in all areas. Signs of vulvovaginal atrophy also were less obvious. When seen 3 months later, the couple reported that their emotional intimacy had improved with the improvement of dyspareunia. However, pain during intercourse was still present, and the patient decided to use 5% lidocaine cream at the "4 o'clock spot" (the most painful area now), if intercourse was to be included.

Improvements in sexual response and lessening of dyspareunia were maintained at 12 months for all three women. Repeated cotton swab testing was not encouraged because the lessening or absence of pain in the sexual situation was the relevant focus.

These three cases illustrate the variable onset of provoked vestibulodynia and the common personality traits that are thought to create stress sufficient to allow sensitization of the pain circuits in women vulnerable to this particular chronic pain syndrome possibly on a genetic basis. Treatment is holistic. In the context of mindfulness practice, women become skillful in recognizing inaccurate thoughts (including catastrophic thoughts) and learn to understand that all thoughts are just mental events, not necessarily truths. Medical adjuncts, including topical treatment with local anesthetics, estriol for postmenopausal women, or mast cell stabilizers (such as cromoglycate), can provide additional benefit. Pain is diminished when intercourse is not obligatory and women sense some control over their situation. It is important to note that as women recover from the pain of provoked vestibulodynia and progress to sexual experiences where they are aroused and have no pain, formal detection of allodynia in an office setting often shows it to still be present but with reduced intensity.

Vaginismus

Obstetrician–gynecologists can manage vaginismus over a series of short visits. The following steps are suggested and have proved helpful, especially for the woman with lifelong vaginismus and unconsummated relationships. It is important to allow the woman control over the pace of therapy and to confirm that she views the endeavor as something she wants for herself, not just for her partner. When this appears not to be the case, referral to a mental health clinician is appropriate, deferring the behavioral approach outlined below. The counseling for vaginismus should include the following steps:

1. The couple should be encouraged to resume sexual activities that exclude any attempt at intercourse. They may need to again have "dates" and specifically and deliberately provide sexual contexts.

2. The reflex contraction of pelvic muscles around the vagina to touch should be explained to the couple, especially when touch has been associated only with negative emotions and physical pain. Women with vaginismus rarely use tampons, avoid the introitus and vagina in sexual play and thus, have had an absence of any neutral sensations from this area of their bodies.

3. Self-touch should be instituted on a daily basis for a few minutes as close to the introitus as possible. This may be done in the bathtub or relaxing on the bed in privacy. This is not sexual, and at first, it will involve high levels of anxiety. However, if the woman engages in this activity daily, the anxiety will quickly lessen.

4. The patient should add imagery to the exercise in item 3, such that she imagines being able to have a limited introital examination, where she could recline on the examina-

tion couch at approximately 70-degree angle so that with the aid of a mirror, she can view the introitus, separate her labia, and be in control of what happens.

5. As soon as the patient is ready, a partial introital examination as in item 4 should be performed. The patient should be encouraged to touch the introitus, moving her finger past the hymen, if possible. Later, the same can be attempted with physician's finger.

6. Once the introitus and vagina have been adequately viewed, a series of vaginal inserts of gradually increasing diameter should be prescribed. An insert is typically left in the vagina for 10–15 minutes while the patient rests comfortably and finds as she reads a book or views television that she is hardly aware of the insert's presence. Plenty of lubrication gel is needed. When symptoms suggestive of provoked vestibulodynia also are present, especially burning with semen ejaculation or dysuria or vulvodynia after intercourse attempts, only the smallest insert should be used before a repeat examination.

7. The examination should be repeated with the patient performing the cotton-swab test for allodynia, if pain has been experienced as opposed to simply feared. Sometimes, the physician can do this, but it is based on the amount of anxiety and apprehension the woman may still have. Her own touching of the introital rim limits the number of false positive results for allodynia.

8. Once larger inserts can be used, the patient should be encouraged to allow her partner to assist her in placing the insert in the vagina.

9. The couple should be encouraged to use the insert briefly during sexual play (to prove to the patient that when her body is physiologically aroused, the insert will still enter the vagina).

10. Once the patient has used the insert on a number of occasions during sexual play, she should be encouraged to insert her partner's penis. It is usually preferable for the woman to be in the same position as when she used the

insert and to hold her partner's penis and insert it herself. He must allow his pelvis to move forward as she tries to insert and both partners gently apply pressure. External lubrication is advised in these first few attempts at penile entry.

Phosphodiesterase inhibitors are useful for temporary situational partner erectile dysfunction that appears at the crucial moment when the woman is finally able to accommodate her partner's penis.

> **CASE NO. 4**. At the first visit, your patient, a 29-year woman and her 30 year-old husband had been married for 7 years but had been unable to consummate their marriage. In addition, the patient was quite hesitant to give direct genital sexual stimulation to her husband, and she has never experienced an orgasm either alone or with him. Because of religious views, the couple abstained from sexual intercourse and direct genital touching without clothes before marriage. The patient recalled enjoying the gentle sensual touching through clothes, but stated that currently, any enjoyment and motivation is brief, perplexing both partners. The patient's whole body, but particularly her thighs tighten when there was penile–vulval contact, and probably there has been no penile–introital contact ever. Although the husband adheres to the patient's wish to avoid vaginal entry, the patient remained hypervigilant that her husband's touches might involve the vaginal opening and that she would be hurt and damaged. She has never explored self-stimulation. She expressed shame about sex and also fears that she may get pregnant despite using birth control pills and condoms. Furthermore, the patient has a number of pain syndromes, including temporomandibular joint pain, marked dysmenorrhea (alleviated by oral contraceptives), frequent headaches, and symptoms compatible with irritable bowel syndrome. The patient's personal history was significant for emotional abuse in childhood, but no physical or sexual abuse. This was the first sexual relationship for both partners.

The initial management included desensitization with self-touch to the introitus and ultimately self-insertion of a vaginal insert. The couple also followed a sensate focus approach with each partner taking turns to give low-key sensual touching and caressing. The partners were encouraged to guide each other. Given the patient's exaggerated thoughts of harm from vaginal entry and fear of pregnancy despite optimal contraception, cognitive therapy was explained, specifically the making of thought records. After 2 months, the patient was used to her own introital touch and felt ready for a partial examination. In the office, she was able to place the smallest vaginal insert through the introitus. Because the insertion was painless, formal cotton-swab testing for provoked vestibulodynia was deferred.

The sensate focus guidelines were gradually relaxed but still any penile–vaginal entry was avoided. The patient continued to check and correct any exaggerated thoughts and made steady progress through the vaginal inserts, including self-insertion and insertion by the husband with the patient's assistance. A further visit allowed a full pelvic examination; no allodynia of provoked vestibulodynia was found.

Intercourse did not follow for some months despite the temporary use of sildenafil by the patient's husband. His gentleness and fear of hurting the patient was part of the difficulty, overcome once the patient practiced using an insert in a "woman superior position." In that position, intercourse proved possible, painless, and enjoyable. Ultimately, sildenafil was discontinued.

The patient's medical history was highly suggestive of vaginismus. Given the clinical overlap between vaginismus and provoked vestibulodynia plus the comorbid temporomandibular joint pain, tension headaches, probable irritable bowel syndrome, the presence of allodynia of provoked vestibulodynia could not be excluded until careful introital examination was possible. Sexual interest/arousal disorder was comorbid and was managed in tandem with vaginismus. The case illustrates how vaginismus is a shared condition, male hesitancy and nonassertiveness being part of the complex dysfunction.

Special Concerns for Older Women

Studies of older women suggest that most older women continue to have sexual interest and response. The two major factors that interfere with these women's sexual lives are lack of a partner or sexual dysfunction in the partner (68). A number of psychologic and biologic factors may influence the sexual lives of older women.

Biologic Factors

Normal genital changes include the following:

- Slower lubrication
- Less vulval swelling
- Reduced length and width of vagina

These changes may lead to pain with vulval stimulation and with penetrative sex, which is not ameliorated by simple lubricants. Longer sexual play and the option of oral or manual stimulation to bring one or both partners to orgasm, if desirable, can be encouraged. When lubricants or moisturizers are inadequate, local estrogen should be considered. After improvement with standard doses, one of the newer ultralow dose preparations may be sufficient.

Normal sexual response changes include the following:

- Slower subjective arousal (and, therefore, taking longer to trigger sexual desire during a given sexual encounter)
- Less need of high arousal or orgasms each time (this can be a problem if both partners are not in agreement and feelings of inadequacy are generated)
- An increased need for affectionate touching that is understood by both partners as not being a prelude to sex

In older women, chronic diseases occur with increasing prevalence. These conditions also have a potential to affect sexual response.

CARDIOVASCULAR DISEASE

Although studies are few, hypertension, its poor control, and the use of β-blockers, are risk factors for all types of sexual dysfunction (185). Comorbid depression is common and is the most likely cause of low sexual desire and arousability in women with ischemic heart disease, although unlike in men, little evidence exists of any direct link to sexual dysfunction.

ARTHRITIS

Pain, debility, reduced mobility, changes to genital tissues found in women with some rheumatic disorders, and comorbid depression may reduce women's sexual response. However, not all studies confirm an increased prevalence of sexual dysfunction. One study of long-term couples in which one partner did or did not have rheumatic disease showed no differences in sexual satisfaction (186). However, the degree of functional impairment was shown to be related to sexual dissatisfaction in both partners. Specifically, the movement needed to participate in intercourse may be precluded or too painful, and sexual caressing and stimulation of self and partner may not be possible because of the involvement of hands and arms. Hip replacement in rheumatoid arthritis was found to improve sexual function to previous levels in 50% of patients (187). Specifically in the context of rheumatoid arthritis, pain, age, and depression have been shown to be the important modulators of women's sexual function (187). Sjögren syndrome can be associated with vaginal dryness, loss of elasticity, and dyspareunia. Systemic sclerosis gives rise to similar symptoms and even ulcerations. These symptoms are difficult to manage and when local lubricants, moisturizers, polymers that attract water, and local estrogen are insufficient, support and encouragement of nonpenetrative sexual activity is necessary.

NEUROLOGIC DISEASE

Usually, neurologic disease leads to sexual deficit, but women with Parkinson disease may experience unwanted hypersexuality when taking dopaminergic agonists. Also severe trauma to the prefrontal lobes or damage to the amygdala in patients with Klüver–Bucy syndrome can lead to a disinhibited hypersexuality. Sometimes the neurologic deficits are ultimately accepted and accommodated, such that women report more intimate sexuality compared with the degree of sexuality before illness. Depression is the most sensitive single predictor of sexual outcome after brain injury, and at least 50% of patients receive the diagnosis of depression after moderate and severe brain injury (188). Brain damage may lead to impaired insight and cognition that interfere with social interaction; sexual relationships may be difficult to begin and maintain. Women whose brain damage has led to hypersexuality are at an increased risk of abuse, coercion, and acquisition of sexually transmitted diseases and unwanted pregnancies. Difficulties with arousal, lubrication, orgasm, and impaired sexual satisfaction and desire occur in 30–88% of women with Parkinson disease, but their attitudes about sexuality and about the disease influence women's sexual functioning more than biomedical factors (189). Sexual dysfunction is common in women with multiple sclerosis. Eventually, 62% of women report loss of genital sensation (190). Contributing factors include fatigue, spasticity, pain, and incontinence. In cases of complete upper motor neuron damage from spinal cord injury, orgasms from usual sexual stimulation are usually lost. However, even when lesions are complete and at any level of the spinal cord, women may experience orgasm from cervical vibrostimulation. It is not clear how this is mediated, although neural supply to the cervix by way of the vagus nerve may be involved (191). When the injury is involving segments below the L-2 nerve, the T-10–L-2 sympathetic outflow from the spinal cord is spared, and this is thought to underlie the retained ability for vaginal congestion and lubrication with mental sexual stimuli. Lower lesions that involve S-2, S-3, and S-4 will preclude any reflex lubrication and any physical sexual sensations from genital stimulation. Cauda equina injuries interrupt autonomic and somatic genital innervation, which precludes genital engorgement, lubrication, sensation, and voluntary control of bladder and bowel. The distress from this can be immense; women with these injuries typically note how they "do not appear to look unwell or have any injury" but have a truly devastating loss. Sexual activity is not without risk for some women with spinal cord injury. Autonomic dysreflexia (acute hypertension from unopposed sympathetic nervous activity) can occur with orgasm in women with lesions above neurologic level T-6. This dangerous consequence is managed with the prophylactic use of calcium channel blockers (192).

DIABETES MELLITUS

Although most studies suggest that rates of low sexual desire are similar in women with and without diabetes, generally difficulties with lubrication are found to be twice as common in women with diabetes, and some, but not all studies, show increased levels of dyspareunia, orgasmic difficulties, and sexual dissatisfaction (193). A strong link exists between dysfunction and comorbid depression. Diabetic control and length of disease do not appear to correlate with the incidence of sexual dysfunction in women, in contrast to the evidence in men. Recent studies have shown metabolic syndrome to be associated with increased sexual dysfunction independent of associated diabetes and obesity. However, this is more marked in premenopausal than postmenopausal women (194). Whether improved management of metabolic syndrome improves sexual function has not been studied.

Psychologic Factors

Older women may be concerned about the safety of sexual activity. They may be concerned that a myocardial infarction or cerebrovascular accident may occur during sexual activity in either partner, especially if there is known disease. Accurate information about the safety of sex should be provided. Patients can be advised that the risk is low and short lasting and that cardiac vascular symptoms are very unlikely if no symptoms arise during exercise testing to six metabolic equivalents (195). Older women also may be afraid of contracting human immunodeficiency virus (HIV). A woman may have had just one lifelong partner so beginning a relationship is new to her. Older women should be counseled about safe sex. Some women experience a lack of sexual attraction. Their marriages may have been arranged or never were based on attraction, the attraction may have faded, or the couples may be together now out of respect, duty, moral reasons, or convenience. Under these circumstances, physicians can explain that sexual wanting and the ability to be aroused together would not be expected to occur on the basis of normal physiology. Many women are relieved to hear that not all couples continue to be sexually active. Changing roles also can be a factor. Women may need care from their partners or may have become the care providers. Difficulties in switching roles may influence sexual relationships. Patients can be counseled or referred for counseling on how to adapt and accept these changes.

Partners

Partners of older women also may be older. Male partners may have erectile dysfunction such that sex becomes focused on unrewarding attempts at intercourse and the mutual pleasure and enjoyment are bypassed—couples move on quickly to intercourse whenever penile firmness allows the attempt. This pattern can continue even when phosphodiesterase inhibitors are prescribed. The couple can be reminded that these medications last many hours, an erection may fade as the male partner's arousal lessens but, unlike erections in the absence of these medications, it can return. The couple can now take their time. Often intercourse has not been possible for some time and the woman may now need local estrogen, at least on a temporary basis (167). Delayed orgasm in male partners can cause prolonged, unrewarding, and increasingly painful intercourse. Currently, this is common with medically enhanced erections, especially from intracavernosal injections whereby the penis is erect but often neither partner is particularly subjectively aroused. It should be explained that erection does not equate with subjective arousal under these circumstances and couples should be encouraged to use other forms of sexual stimulation in addition to the act of intercourse. Also, men may not experience orgasms every time they use erectile enhancement—older men have orgasm less frequently than middle-aged men. Alternatively, the woman's partner (male or female) may be much younger than she, and desire discrepancy needs to be negotiated.

Special Concerns for Patients With Cancer

Difficulties in sexual function subsequent to breast cancer treatment are the most likely areas of distress to persist beyond 1 year after diagnosis. Sexual self-image can be negatively affected, and there may be fear of recurrence causing hesitancy to start a new relationship. The need to disclose the medical details and fear of rejection may act as deterrents. The stress and sadness of possible imposed infertility may further lessen self-image and sexual desire. However, many studies conclude that major negative factors that affect sexual response are chemotherapy that leads to premature menopause and the use of aromatase inhibitors (196, 197). Treatment of vulvovaginal atrophy and menopausal symptoms with systemic estrogen is almost always contraindicated and local estrogen also is officially contraindicated, but many health care providers prescribe it sparingly when conservative nonhormonal regimes fail to alleviate dyspareunia and the couple chooses not to limit themselves to nonpenetrative sex. In one report, hyaluronic acid vaginal gel was shown to improve symptoms in 85% of women, comparable with women who received vaginal estriol (166). The use of estradiol, 10 micrograms twice weekly, and the estradiol vaginal ring results in serum levels of 4.6 pg/mL and 8 pg/mL. Women who use aromatase inhibitors and vaginal estrogen may show a small increase in serum estradiol levels (198); a prospective trial of aromatase inhibition plus vaginal estrogen is underway. Investigational vaginal DHEA that appears not to increase serum levels of testosterone or estrogen has not been studied in breast cancer patients but appears promising. Intravaginal testosterone may alleviate symptoms (196), but any systemic absorption could increase serum estrogen through aromatization. Research in lesbian and bisexual women with breast cancer histories is beginning. A case–control study confirmed similar predictors of sexual function to those of heterosexual women: a sense of sexual attractiveness, paucity of urogynecological symptoms, postmenopausal status, and relationship harmony (199).

Gynecologic cancer, and especially its treatment, can have marked, mostly negative effects, on women's sexual well-being in terms of their sense of femininity, self-image, confidence, sense of desirability, misgivings as to the etiologic role of past sexual activities and on women's sexual function from the treatment-related anatomic and hormonal changes (200).

Relationships with supportive partners have a strong positive effect on women's sexual well-being and their ability to cope with the imposed sexual changes.

Loss of sexual organs from surgery and ovarian function and fertility from chemotherapy, interference with vulval and vaginal congestion from damaged autonomic nerves in radical hysterectomy, and tissue damage from radiation therapy—especially vaginal agglutination—may all contribute to the sexual changes. Radical hysterectomy for cervical cancer has been noted to have persistent negative effects on sexual desire, whereas difficulty with lubrication may lessen over time if, as noted in one study, the autonomic nerves in the cardinal and uterosacral ligaments are spared (201). Some research suggests that more marked sexual dysfunction in women with cervical cancer compared with controls is seen in those with a history of sexual abuse (81). Resumption of intercourse is not necessarily an indicator of satisfaction with sexual intimacy because some couples may engage only to keep or satisfy their partners (81). A systematic review examined 34 articles outlining sexual concerns (202). Research is minimal on the sexual well-being of lesbian women with gynecologic cancer; there is evidence of differences in communication, resolution of conflict as well as less focus on vaginal penetration in nonheterosexual relationships (200).

Because most women who receive radiation therapy are at risk of developing vaginal agglutination and stenosis within the first 3 months of therapy, vaginal insert treatment is important, and measures to increase adherence require urgent study. Reliving the invasiveness and trauma of their treatment, embarrassment, and reminding women of the cancer are cited as barriers, whereas seeing dilator use as an integral extension of treatment and recovery can help adherence (203). Local estrogen also can be given. Preliminary study of mindfulness training incorporated into a psychoeducational program for women with arousal disorder subsequent to gynecologic cancer showed benefit (144, 204). Pretreatment sexual assessment and advice, repeated at 3 months after treatment has been shown to allow healthier sexual well-being and function compared with standard pretreatment information and nursing care (205).

CASE NO. 5. A 57-year old patient reported total loss of sexual desire, reduced arousal, and rubbing and burning dyspareunia only partially remedied by external lubricant, all since stopping her systemic estrogen and progesterone 2 years previously when breast cancer was diagnosed. Lumpectomy and radiation therapy were followed by tamoxifen. Her mood had been stable, and the relationship with her husband remained positive despite sexual infrequency and her lack of sexual enjoyment. The patient previously received compounded HT from her naturopath and planned to restart it despite her oncologist's advice to the contrary.

The reflex response to attribute sexual changes to one factor, especially a medical one, is common. The timing of dysfunction coincided with cessation of HT, diagnosis and treatment of breast cancer, and possibly other unrelated contextual factors. In the area of sexual medicine, it is usually the person with the disease rather than the disease itself that is most important in assessment and treatment. Further inquiry clarified that, in this patient's view, the decreased hormone production, lessened energy, cancer diagnosis, and dyspareunia implied that she was aging. Similarly, any move to nonpenetrative sex and cutting back on her workload would imply being generally and sexually substandard, and therefore, unattractive.

The stance that her lost desire must all be due to hormonal lack gradually faded as the patient recounted other coincident major stressors in her life. During sexual encounters, she worried about the pain from intercourse and that she was old and less feminine. Moderate vulvovaginal atrophy was present on physical examination; there was no allodynia typical of provoked vestibulodynia. Pelvic muscle tone was within normal limits.

The sexual response cycle was explained, including the need to be present and attend to sexual stimulation that could potentially trigger arousal and desire. The couple was encouraged first to address the patient's work volume. Then, ways to manage stress were discussed, including mindfulness techniques. It was suggested that sexual encounters could be planned, should not take place late at night, and could involve partners taking turns in low-key sensual touching and caressing. The patient began to reduce her workload, and to help reduce stress, both partners started to practice mindfulness. When seen 3 months later, the couple reported excellent sexual experiences without pain and with arousal pleasure and orgasm.

The patient's diagnoses were sexual interest/arousal disorder and dyspareunia. The major etiologic factor was the distraction related to family and work issues, compounding stress from the breast cancer diagnosis and treatment and its detrimental effect on the patient's self-image. Moderate vulvovaginal atrophy and lack of arousal contributed to the dyspareunia. Although estrogen deficit was obvious on examination, the poor correlation between visual changes and symptoms encouraged deferring the controversial question of local estrogen treatment. Once stressors were deliberately reduced and mindfulness practice instituted, adequate sexual arousal and a use of a simple lubricant allowed painless intercourse.

Complementary and Alternative Medicine

Alternative therapies for sexual dysfunction can be classified into one of the two categories:

1. Products that promote genital blood flow
2. Products that promote sexual desire

It is necessary to ask patients if they are using alternative products for any sexual difficulties, clarify the lack of efficacy and safety data, and also assess and manage patients' sexual difficulties in as safe a manner as possible.

Products That Promote Genital Blood Flow

A small number of products containing arginine are marketed to promote genital blood flow. Nitric oxide is produced from arginine, but no evidence exists that it is the lack of substrate that underlies problematic vulval and vaginal nitric oxide-mediated smooth muscle relaxation. One study showed improvement in sexual function from an arginine-containing nutritional supplement in premenopausal but not in postmenopausal women (206). A scientific study that used genital MRI and visual sexual stimuli disproved reduced genital congestion in women with arousal disorder and showed comparable increases in genital congestion from sildenafil and from placebo (207). The previously noted degree of disconnection between genital events and subjective arousal must be kept in mind when considering usefulness of directly acting genital vasodilators. Without scientific study, gingko biloba is promoted as increasing genital blood flow. Caution is particularly needed regarding interaction with anticoagulants and also regarding reports of contamination of some brands of gingko biloba with colchicine.

Products That Promote Sexual Desire, Arousal, Orgasm, and Sexual Satisfaction

A botanical mixture of borage seed oil, evening primrose oil, *coleus forskohlii* extract, and angelica root extract has been studied in an RCT. A modest benefit over placebo was noted in women with desire, arousal, and orgasm dysfunction in that desire and arousal but not lubrication showed statistically significant benefit on some of the measures used. However, overall satisfaction with sexual life, number of successful encounters, and sexual distress did not improve (208).

As previously mentioned, oral DHEA in varying forms of purity and potency is readily available in the United States, and its use is not evidence-based (105). A number of other products, usually mixtures that may contain testosterone, are available, especially in Chinese herbal preparations. However, no scientific evidence exists of their efficacy or safety.

Future Directions in Research and Therapy

Recent qualitative research confirms that an overlap exists between sexual arousal and desire. This, along with brain imaging of sexual arousal, emphasizes the complexity of sexual arousal and desire. Clinical research continues to link women's desire and arousal to mental health and psychosocial factors. Nevertheless, attempts have been made to find a molecule to repair women's sexual dysfunction. Two trials of nonhormonal medications (flibanserin and bremelanotide) were discontinued. A different sponsor is conducting the clinical trial of the latter agent with nasal or subcutaneous administration in an attempt to improve safety. The trials of a testosterone gel were completed and showed no benefit over placebo (114). Although pursuit of a "quick fix" by industry may well continue, the focus may now move to more structured manual psychologic treatments, which can be used by multiple clinicians, adapted for different patient populations and cultures, and suitable for therapy in small-group format, and possibly aided by Internet access. Similarly, the management of chronic dyspareunia from provoked vestibulodynia is increasingly recognized as requiring an interdisciplinary biopsychosexual approach and the protocols are modified as more is learned about brain processing of chronic pain conditions and modulation of the these networks by psychologic and pharmacologic means. In particular, the modality of mindfulness is being increasingly incorporated into treatment of sexual dysfunctions in general and into management of chronic pain, including that from provoked vestibulodynia.

Regarding pharmacologic therapy, given the robust evidence of an association between mood and sexual desire and arousal, sexually neutral antidepressants, such as agomelatine, are needed. Further research of the reported sexual benefit from vaginal DHEA is ongoing. Selective estrogen receptor modulators (SERMs) with estrogen activity in the vulva and vagina could provide sexual benefit and also improve bone, vascular endothelium, and brain health, while maintaining estrogen receptor antagonism or neutrality in the breast and endometrium. To date, SERMs have some class effects but also individual effects; for example, ospemifene has been shown to ameliorate vaginal atrophy and improve dyspareunia (209). Tissue selective estrogen complexes combine a SERM with estrogen in an attempt to provide optimal results for their blended tissue activity. A combination of a SERM (bazedoxifene) plus conjugated estrogens is under clinical study and has been shown to improve vulvovaginal atrophy and reduce bone loss while showing a neutral effect on breast and endometrium (210).

Conclusions

When women experience sexual symptoms, the underlying problems may not be intrinsically sexual, and dealing with the basic psychologic issues often allows the sexual symptoms "to take care of themselves." However, women frequently believe the issues to be primarily sexual and wish to discuss them with the gynecologist rather than with a psychologist or a psychiatrist. It is the obstetrician–gynecologist's role to clarify with a patient that the issues have a global psychologic nature. A psychologic referral may be needed as the first step in the patient's management. The large number of women who lose sexual motivation and satisfaction subsequent to provoked vestibulodynia or estrogen-related vulvovaginal atrophy, including women with gynecologic and breast cancer, necessitates obstetrician–gynecologists' ability to carefully assess sexual pain and dysfunction. When even low-dose vaginal estrogen is not considered safe because of a history of breast cancer, sensitivity and skill are needed to assist the woman and her partner to adapt to non-penetrative sex. Obstetrician–gynecologists should be aware of a strong link between depression and sexual dysfunction in the context of chronic gynecologic and nongynecologic disease. Moreover, despite inherent risk of medication-associated sexual dysfunction, achieving remission of depression is the mainstay of treatment of the sexual dysfunction.

Resources

American College of Obstetricians and Gynecologists. WebTreats: sex and sexuality. Washington, DC: American College of Obstetricians and Gynecologists; 2013. Available at: www.acog.org/About_ACOG/ACOG_Departments/Resource_Center/WEBTREATS_Sex_and_Sexuality. Retrieved January 16, 2014.

The following list is for information purposes only. Referral to these sources and web sites does not imply the endorsement of the American College of Obstetricians and Gynecologists. This list is not meant to be comprehensive. The exclusion of a source or web site does not reflect the quality of that source of web site. Please note that web sites are subject to change without notice.

Publications

Fruhauf S, Gerger H, Maren Schmidt H, Munder T, Barth J. Efficacy of psychological interventions for sexual dysfunction: a systematic review and meta-analysis. Arch Sex Behav 2013;42:915–33.

Heiman JR, LoPiccolo J. Becoming orgasmic: a sexual and personal growth program for women. rev. & expanded ed. New York (NY): Prentice Hall; 1987.

Organizations

American Association of Sexuality Educators, Counselors and Therapists
1444 I Street, NW Suite 700
Washington, DC 20005
Web: www.aasect.org
Telephone: 202-216-9646

American Psychological Association
Aging and Human Sexuality Resource Guide
750 First St., NE
Washington, DC 20002-4242
Web: www.apa.org/pi/aging/resources/guides/sexuality.aspx
Telephone: 800-374-2721

International Society for the Study of Women's Sexual Health
Two Woodfield Lake
1100E. Woodfield Road, Suite 350
Schaumburg, IL 60173
Web: www.isswsh.org
Telephone: 847-517-7225

National Vulvodynia Association
PO Box 4491
Silver Spring, MD 20914-4491
Web: www.nva.org
Telephone: 301-299-0775

(continued)

Resources *(continued)*

North American Menopause Society
5900 Landerbrook Dr., Suite 390
Mayfield Heights, OH 44124
Web: www.menopause.org
Telephone: 440-442-7550

Sexuality Information and Education Council of the United States
90 John Street, Suite 402
New York, NY 10038
Web: www.siecus.org
Telephone: 212-819-9770

Society for Sex Therapy and Research
6311 W. Gross Point Rd.
Niles, IL 60714
Web: www.sstarnet.org
Telephone: 847-647-8832

The Kinsey Institute
Indiana University
Morrison 313
1165 E. Third St
Bloomington, IN 47405
Web: www.indiana.edu/~kinsey
Telephone: 812-855-7686

Test Your Clinical Skills

Complete the answer sheet at the back of this book and return it to the American College of Obstetricians and Gynecologists to receive Continuing Medical Education credits. The answers appear on page 102.

Directions: Select the one best answer or completion.

1. In a study of 589 pregnant women what percentage of women excluded sexual intercourse by the third trimester?
   A.   15
   B.   33
   C.   40
   D.   60

2. A woman's dissatisfaction with her sexual relationship at 1 year postpartum can be predicted by sexual inactivity as early as at
   A.   8 weeks postpartum
   B.   12 weeks of gestation
   C.   24 weeks of gestation
   D.   32 weeks of gestation

3. In a web-based survey of women deemed to be sexually functional, what proportion of women reported limiting sexual activity to when they felt sexual desire at the outset?
   A.   15%
   B.   25%
   C.   50%
   D.   75%

4. A woman who refers to herself as a "wasbian" is probably in transition to which sexual orientation?
   A.   Asexual
   B.   Bisexual
   C.   Heterosexual
   D.   Homosexual

5. In the female sexual response, vaginal congestion is mostly mediated by which substance?
   A. Calcitonin gene-related peptide
   B. Helospectin
   C. Substance P
   D. Vasoactive intestinal polypeptide

6. Compared with women with intact ovaries, women who have had bilateral oophorectomy have increased rates of
   A. reports of low desire
   B. distress over low desire
   C. problems with orgasm
   D. orientation changes

7. In summarizing the studies on testosterone treatment, the author concludes that
   A. testosterone was studied in clinical trials in women who have testosterone deficiency
   B. testosterone patch and testosterone gel studies found increased desire from active drug
   C. women in the trials typically reported one or less than one satisfactory sexual experience per month at baseline
   D. testosterone is not approved for use in women in the United States and although it is approved in Europe, it is no longer marketed there

8. Mindfulness-based cognitive therapy
   A. is a subtype of sex therapy
   B. reduces pain and sexual dysfunction from provoked vestibulodynia
   C. improves sexual dysfunction in women without gyne-cologic cancer but not those with gynecologic cancer
   D. is a traditional cognitive-based therapy but adds an optional meditation practice

9. The author suggests that self-stimulation may be helpful for patients with which psychologic factor?
   A. Fear of closeness
   B. Fear of losing control
   C. Fear of loss of relationship
   D. Lack of trust of others

10. Which of the following is not part of holistic therapy for provoked vestibulodynia?
    A. Education on the pathophysiology of provoked vestibulodynia
    B. Learning the role of stress in provoked vestibulodynia
    C. Goal of penetrative sex within 3 months
    D. Learning that thoughts are not truths

11. Of the three case studies of provoked vestibulodynia how many women were able to achieve sexual penetration after 6 months of treatment?
    A. 0
    B. 1
    C. 2
    D. 3

12. Hypersexuality is a recognized complication of
    A. arthritis
    B. brain damage
    C. diabetes
    D. metabolic syndrome

13. Elective bilateral oophorectomy in middle-aged premenopausal women who require hysterectomy for benign disease is associated with
    A. no changes in sexual function or desire when followed for up to 3 years
    B. reduced desire when compared with women with retained ovaries
    C. reduced orgasm when compared with women with retained ovaries
    D. reduced genital sensation when compared with women with retained ovaries

14. In the largest and longest study of women who undergo menopause, desire and sexual response were most influenced by
    A. age at menopause
    B. estrogen status
    C. women's feelings for their partners
    D. years since the last menstrual period

References

1. Naeinian MR, Shaeiri MR, Hosseini FS. General health and quality of life in patients with sexual dysfunctions. J Urol 2011;8:127–31. (Level II-3)

2. U.S. Department of Health and Human Services. The Surgeon General's call to action to promote sexual health and responsible sexual behavior. Washington, DC: U.S. Department of Health and Human Services; 2001. Available at http://surgeongeneral.gov/library/sexualhealth/call.pdf. Retrieved January 6, 2014. (Level III)

3. Santoro N, Komi J. Prevalence and impact of vaginal symptoms among post-menopausal women. J Sex Med 2009;6:2133–42. (Level II-3)

4. Nappi RE, Kokot-Kierepa M. Women's voices in the menopause: results from an international survey on vaginal atrophy. Maturitas 2010;67:233–8. (Level III)

5. Burri A, Spector T. Recent and lifelong sexual dysfunction in a female UK population sample: prevalence and risk factors. J Sex Med 2011;8:2420–30. (Level II-3)

6. Pujols Y, Seal BN, Meston CM. The association between sexual satisfaction and body image in women [published erratum appears in J Sex Med 2010;7:2295]. J Sex Med 2010;7:905–16. (Level II-3)

7. Hartmann U, Philippsohn S, Heiser K, Ruffer-Hesse C. Low sexual desire in midlife and older women: personality factors, psychosocial development, present sexuality. Menopause 2004;11:726–40. (Level III)

8. Maserejian NN, Shifren JL, Parish J, Braunstein GD, Gerstenberger EP, Rosen RC. The presentation of hypoactive sexual desire disorder in pre-menopausal women. J Sex Med 2010;7:3439–48. (Level II-3)

9. Ferenidou K, Kapoteli V, Moisidis K, Koutsogiannis I, Giakoumelos A, Hatzichristou D. Presence of a sexual problem may not affect women's satisfaction from their sexual function. J Sex Med 2008;5:631–9. (Level III)

10. Shifren JL, Monz BU, Russo PA, Segreti A, Johannes CB. Sexual problems and distress in United States women: prevalence and correlates. Obstet Gynecol 2008;112:970–8. (Level II-3)

11. Dennerstein L, Guthrie JR, Hayes RD, DeRogatis LR, Lehert P. Sexual function, dysfunction, and sexual distress in a prospective, population-based sample of mid-aged, Australian-born women. J Sex Med 2008;5:2291–9. (Level III)

12. Althof SE, Dean J, Derogatis LR, Rosen RC, Sisson M. Current perspectives on the clinical assessment and diagnosis of female sexual dysfunction and clinical studies of potential therapies: statement of concern. J Sex Med 2005; 2(suppl):146–53. (Level III)

13. King M, Holt V, Nazareth I. Women's view of their sexual difficulties: agreement and disagreement for the clinical diagnoses. Arch Sex Behav 2007;36:281–8. (Level II-3)

14. Cain VS, Johannes CB, Avis NE, Mohr B, Schocken M, Skurnick J, et al. Sexual functioning and practices in a multi-ethnic study of mid-life women: baseline results from SWAN. J Sex Res 2003;40:266–76. (Level II-3)

15. Laumann EO, Nicolosi A, Glasser DB, Paik A, Gingell C, Moreira, et al. Sexual problems among women and men aged 40-80 y: prevalence and correlates identified in the Global Study of Sexual Attitudes and Behaviours. GSSAB Investigators' Group. Int J Impot Res 2005;17:39–57. (Level II-3)

16. West SL, D'Aloisio AA, Agans RP, Kalsbeek WD, Borisov NN, Thorp JM. Prevalence of low sexual desire and hypoactive sexual desire disorder in a nationally representative sample of US women. Arch Intern Med 2008;168: 1441–9. (Level II-3)

17. Addis IB, Van Den Eeden SK, Wassel-Fyr CL,Vittinghoff E, Bown JS, Thom DH. Sexual activity and function in middle-aged and older women. Reproductive Risk Factors for Incontinence Study at Kaiser Study Group. Obstet Gynecol 2006;107:755–64. (Level II-3)

18. Bancroft J, Loftus J, Long JS. Distress about sex: A national survey of women in heterosexual relationships. Arch Sex Behav 2003;32:193–208. (Level III)

19. Laumann EO, Paik A, Rosen RC. Sexual dysfunction in the United States: prevalence and predictors [published erratum appears in JAMA 1999;281:1174]. JAMA 1999;281:537–44. (Level II-3)

20. Danielsson I, Sjoberg I, Stelund H, Wikman M. Prevalence and incidence of prolonged and severe dyspareunia in women: results from a population study. Scand J Public Health 2003;31:113–8. (Level II-3)

21. Laumann EO, Waite LJ. Sexual dysfunction among older adults: prevalence and risk factors from a nationally representative U.S. probability sample of men and women 57-85 years of age. J Sex Med 2008;5:2300–11. (Level II-3)

22. Lindau ST, Schumm LP, Laumann EO, Levinson W, O'Muircheartaigh CA, Waite LJ. A study of sexuality and health among older adults in the United States. N Engl J Med 2007;357:762–74. (Level II-3)

23. Kingsberg SA, Wysocki S, Magnus L, Krychman ML. Vulvar and vaginal atrophy in postmenopausal women: Findings from the REVIVE (REal Women's VIews of Treatment Options for Menopausal Vaginal ChangEs) survey. J Sex Med 2013;10:1790–9. (Level II-3)

24. Van Geelen JM, van de Weijer PH, Arnolds HT. Urogenital symptoms and resulting discomfort in non-institutionalized Dutch women aged 50-75 years. Int Urogynecol J Pelvic Floor Dysfunct 2000;11:9–14. (Level II-3)

25. Nichols M. Sexual fuction in women with women; lesbians and lesbian relationships. In: Goldstein I, Meston CM, Davis SR, Traish AM, editors. Women's sexual function and dysfunction: study, diagnosis, and treatment. London: Taylor & Francis; 2006. p. 307–14. (Level III)

26. Armstrong H, Reissing E. Chronic vulvo-vaginal pain in lesbian, bisexual and other sexual minority women [abstract]. J Sex Med 2012;9(suppl 3):166. (Level III)

27. Shindel AW, Rowen TS, Lin TC, Li CS, Robertson PA, Breyer BN. An Internet survey of demographic and health factors associated with risk of sexual dys-

function in women who have sex with women. J Sex Med 2012;9:1261–71. (Level II-3)

28. Klein C, Gorzalka BB. Sexual functioning in transsexuals following hormone therapy and genital surgery: a review. J Sex Med 2009;11:2922–39; quiz 2940–1. (Level III)

29. Moel JE, Buttner MM, O'Hara MW, Stuart S, Gorman L. Sexual function in the postpartum period: effects of maternal depression and interpersonal psychotherapy treatment. Arch Womens Ment Health 2010;13:495–504. (Level I)

30. Erol B, Sanli O, Korkmaz D, Seyhan A, Akman T, Kadioglu A. A cross-sectional study of female sexual function and dysfunction during pregnancy. J Sex Med 2007;4:1381–7. (Level II-3)

31. Signorello LB, Harlow BL, Chekos AK, Repke JT. Postpartum sexual functioning and its relationship to perineal trauma: a restrospective cohort study of primiparous women. Am J Obstet Gynecol 2001;184:881–8; discussion 888–90. (Level II-3)

32. Radestad I, Olsson A, Nissen E, Rubertsson C. Tears in the vagina, perineum, sphincter ani, and rectum and first sexual intercourse after childbirth: a nationwide follow-up. Birth 2008;35:98–106. (Level II-3)

33. Gordon B, Mackrodt C, Fern E, Truesdale A, Ayers S, Grant A. The Ipswich Childbirth Study: 1. A randomized evaluation of two stage postpartum perineal repair leaving the skin unsutured. Br J Obstet Gynaecol 1998;105: 435–40. (Level I)

34. Citak N, Cam C, Arslan H, Karateke A, Tug N, Ayaz R, et al. Postpartum sexual function of women and the effects of early pelvic floor muscle exercises. Acta Obstet Gynecol Scand 2010;89:817–22. (Level I)

35. DeJudicibus MA, McCabe MP. Psychological factors and the sexuality of pregnant and postpartum women. J Sex Res 2002;39:94–103. (Level II-3)

36. van Brummen HJ, Bruinse HW, van de Pol G, Heintz AP, van der Vaart CH. Which factors determine the sexual function 1 year after childbirth? BJOG 2006;113:914–8. (Level II-3)

37. Dennerstein L, Dudley E, Burger H. Are changes in sexual functioning during mid-life due to aging or menopause? Fertil Steril 2001;76:456–60. (Level II-3)

38. Avis NE, Stellato R, Crawford S, Johannes C, Longcope C. Is there an association between menopause status and sexual functioning? Menopause 2000;7:297–309. (Level II-3)

39. Woods NF, Mitchell ES, Smith-Di Julio K. Sexual desire during the menopausal transition and early postmenopause: observations from the Seattle Midlife Women's Health Study. J Women's Health (Larchmt) 2010;19: 209–18. (Level II-3)

40. Birnbaum GE, Cohen O, Wertheimer V. It is all about intimacy? Age, menopausal status, and women's sexuality. Pers Relatsh 2007;14:167–85. (Level III)

41. van der Stege JG, Groen H, van Zadelhoff SJ, Lambalk CB, Braat DD, van Kasteren YM, et al. Decreased androgen concentrations and diminished

general and sexual well-being in women with premature ovarian failure. Menopause 2008; 15:23–31. (Level II-3)

42. Leiblum SR, Koochaki PE, Rodenberg CA, Barton IP, Rosen RC. Hypoactive sexual desire disorder in postmenopausal women: US results from the Women's International Study of Health and Sexuality (WISHeS). Menopause 2006;13:46–56. (Level II-3)

43. Dennerstein L, Koochaki P, Barton I, Graziottin A. Hypoactive sexual desire disorder in menopausal women: a survey of western European women. J Sex Med 2006;3:212–22. (Level II-3)

44. Teplin V, Vittinghoff E, Lin F, Learman LA, Richter HE, Kuppermann M. Oophorectomy in premenopausal women: health-related quality of life and sexual functioning. Obstet Gynecol 2007;109:347–54. (Level II-2)

45. Wierman ME, Basson R, Davis SR, Khosla S, Miller K, Rosner W, et al. Androgen therapy in women: an Endocrine Society Clinical Practice Guideline. J Clin Endocrinol Metab 2006;1:3697–710. (Level III)

46. Stephenson KR, Ahrold TK, Meston CM. The association between sexual motives and sexual satisfaction: gender differences and categorical comparisons. Arch Sex Behav 2011;40:607–18. (Level II-3)

47. Meston CM, Hamilton LD, Harte CB. Sexual motivation in women as a function of age [published erratum appears in J Sex Med 2010; 7:3803]. J Sex Med 2009;6:3305–19. (Level II-3)

48. McCall K, Meston C. Differences between pre- and postmenopausal women in cues for sexual desire. J Sex Med 2007;4:364–71.

49. Carvalheira AA, Brotto LA, Leal I. Women's motivations for sex: exploring the diagnostic and statistical manual, 4th edition, text revision criteria for hypoactive sexual desire and female sexual arousal disorders. J Sex Med 2010;7:1454–63. (Level II-3)

50. Goldhammer DL, McCabe MP. A qualitative exploration of the meaning and experience of sexual desire among partnered women. Can J Hum Sex 2011;20:19–34. (Level III)

51. Laan E, Both S. What makes women experience desire? Fem Psychol 2008;18:505–14. (Level III)

52. Sidi H, Naing L, Midin M, Nik Jaafar NR. The female sexual response cycle: do Malaysian women conform to the circular model? J Sex Med 2008;5:2359–66. (Level III)

53. American Psychiatric Association. Diagnostic and statistical manual of mental disorders: DSM-V. 5th ed. Washington, DC: APA; 2013. Available at: http://www.dsm5.org/Pages/Default.aspx. Retrieved January 14, 2014. (Level III)

54. Basson R. A model of women's sexual arousal. J Sex Marital Ther 2002;28:1–10. (Level III)

55. Brotto LA. The DSM diagnostic criteria for hypoactive sexual desire disorder in women. Arch Sex Behav 2010;39:221–39. (Level III)

56. Graham CA. The DSM diagnostic criteria for female sexual arousal disorder. Arch Sex Behav 2010;39:240–55. (Level III)

57. Chivers ML, Seto MC, Lalumiere ML, Laan E, Grimbos T. Agreement of self-reported and genital measures of sexual arousal in men and women: a meta-analysis. Arch Sex Behav 2010;39:5–56. (Meta-analysis)

58. Laan E, van Driel EM, van Lunsen RH. Genital responsiveness in healthy women with and without sexual arousal disorder. J Sex Med 2008;5:1424–35. (Level III)

59. Arnow BA, Millheiser L, Garrett A, Lake Polan M, Glover GH, Hill KR, et al. Women with hypoactive sexual desire disorder compared to normal females: a functional magnetic resonance imaging study. Neuroscience 2009;158:484–502. (Level III)

60. Sanders SA, Graham CA, Milhausen RR. Predicting sexual problems in women: the relevance of sexual excitation and sexual inhibition. Arch Sex Behav 2008;37:241–51. (Level II-3)

61. de Jong DC. The role of attention in sexual arousal: implications for treatment of sexual dysfunction. J Sex Res 2009;46:237–48. (Level III)

62. Carvalho J, Nobre P. Sexual desire in women: an integrative approach regarding psychological, medical, and relationship dimensions. J Sex Med 2010;7:1807–15. (Level II-3)

63. Carvalho J, Nobre P. Predictors of women's sexual desire: the role of psychopathology, cognitive-emotional determinants, relationship dimensions, and medical factors. J Sex Med 2010;7:928–37. (Level II-3)

64. Nobre PJ, Pinto-Gouveia J. Cognitions, emotions, and sexual response: analysis of the relationship among automatic thoughts, emotional responses, and sexual arousal. Arch Sex Behav 2008;37:652–61. (Level II-3)

65. ter Kuille MM, Both S, van Uden J. The effects of experimentally-induced sad and happy mood on sexual arousal in sexually healthy women. J Sex Med 2010;7:1177–84. (Level III)

66. Oliveira C, Nobre PJ. Cognitive structures in women with sexual dysfunction: the role of early maladaptive schemas. J Sex Med 2013;10:1755–63. (Level II-3)

67. Heiman JR, Talley DR, Bailen JL, Okin TA, Rosenberg SJ, Pace CR, et al. Sexual function and satisfaction in heterosexual couples when men are administered sildenafil citrate (Viagra) for erectile dysfunction: a multicentre, randomized, double-blind, placebo-controlled trial. BJOG 2007;114:437–47. (Level I)

68. Fugl-Meyer K, Fugl-Meyer AR. Sexual disabilities are not singularities. Int J Impot Res 2002;14:487–93. (Level II-3)

69. Janssen E, Everaerd W, Spiering M, Janssen J. Automatic processes and the appraisal of sexual stimuli: toward an information processing model of sexual arousal. J Sex Res 2000;37:8–23. (Level III)

70. Lauman E, Gagnon J, Michael RT, Michaels S, editors. The social organization of sexuality: sexual practices in the United States. Chicago (IL): University of Chicago Press; 1994. (Level III)

71. Diamond L. Was it a phase? Young women's relinquishment of lesbian/bi-sexual identities over a 5 year period. J Personality and Soc Psychol 2003; 84:352–364. (Level III)

72. Diamond LM. The desire disorder in research on sexual orientation in women: contributions of dynamic systems theory. Arch Sex Behav 2012; 41:73–83. (Level III)

73. Vrangalova Z, Savin-Williams RC. Mostly heterosexual and mostly gay/lesbian: evidence for new sexual orientation identities. Arch Sex Behav 2012;41:85–101. (Level II-3)

74. Ehrstrom S, Kornfeld D, Rylander E, Bohm-Starke N. Chronic stress in women with localised provoked vulvodynia. J Psychosom Obstet Gynaecol 2009;30:73–9. (Level II-3)

75. Basson R. The recurrent pain and sexual sequelae of provoked vestibulo-dynia: a perpetuating cycle. J Sex Med 2012;9:2077–92. (Level III)

76. Hamann S, Herman RA, Nolan CL, Wallen K. Men and women differ in amygdala response to visual sexual stimuli. Nat Neurosci 2004;7:411–6. (Level III)

77. Mani SK, Allen JM, Clark JH, Blaustein JD, O'Malley BW. Convergent path-ways for steroid hormone-and neurotransmitter-induced rat sexual behav-ior [published erratum appears in Science 1995;268:1833]. Science 1994; 265:1246–48. (Animal study)

78. Blaustein JD. Progestin receptors: neuronal integrators of hormonal and environmental stimulation. Ann N Y Acad Sci 2003;1007:238–50. (Level III)

79. Segraves RT, Clayton A, Crift H, Wolf A, Warnock J. Buproprion sustained release for the treatment of hypoactive sexual desire disorder in premeno-pausal women. J Clin Psychopharmacol 2004;24:339–42. (Level I)

80. Dennerstein L, Lehert P, Guthrie J. The effects of the menopausal transi-tion and biopsychosocial factors on well-being. Arch Women Ment Health 2002;5:15–22.

81. Bergmark K, Avall-Lundqvist E, Dickman PW, Henningsohn L, Steineck G. Vaginal changes and sexuality in women with a history of cervical cancer. N Engl J Med 1999;340:1383–9. (Level II-3)

82. Bekker MD, Hogewoning CR, Wallner C, Elzevier HW, DeRuiter MC. The somatic and autonomic innervation of the clitoris; preliminary evidence of sexual dysfunction after minimally invasive slings. J Sex Med 2012;9: 1566–78. (Level III)

83. Salonia A, Giraldi A, Chivers ML, Georgiadis JR, Levin R, Maravilla KR, et al. Physiology of women's sexual function: basic knowledge and new find-ings. J Sex Med 2010;7:2637–60. (Level III)

84. Shih C, Cold CJ, Yang CC. Cutaneous corpuscular receptors of the human glans clitoris: descriptive characteristics and comparison with the glans penis. J Sex Med 2013;10:1783–9. (Level III)

85. Modelska K, Litwack S, Ewing SK, Yaffe K. Endogenous estrogen levels affect sexual function in elderly post-menopausal women. Maturitas 2004; 49:124–33. (Level II-3)

86. Laan E, Van Lunsen RH. Hormones and sexuality in postmenopausal women: a psychophysiological study. J Psychom Obstet Gynaecol 1997;18: 126–33. (Level III)

87. Maravilla KR, HeimanJR, Garland PA,Cao Y, Carter WO, Peterson BT, et al. Dynamic MR imaging of the sexual arousal response in women. J Sex Marital Ther 2003;29(suppl):71–6. (Level III)

88. Freedman MA. Vaginal pH, estrogen, and genital atrophy. Menopause Management 2008;17:9–13.

89. Kao A, Binik Y, Amsel R, Funaro D, Leroux N, Khalife S. Biopsychosocial predictors of postmenopausal dyspareunia: the role of steroid hormones, vulvovaginal atrophy, cognitive-emotional factors and dyadic adjustment. J Sex Med 2012;9:2066–76.

90. Bradshaw HB, Berkley KJ. Estrogen replacement reverses ovariectomy-induced vaginal hyperalgesia in the rat. Maturitas 2002;41:157–65. (Animal study)

91. Bachmann GA, Leiblum SR. Sexuality in sexagenarian women. Maturitas 1991;13:43–50. (Level III)

92. Gorodeski GI. Aging and estrogen effects on transcervical-transvaginal epithelial permeability. J Clin Endocrinol Metab 2005;90:345–51. (Level III)

93. Lara LA, Useche B, Ferriani RA, Reis RM, de Sa MF, de Freaitas MM, et al. The effects of hypoestrogenism on the vaginal wall: interference with the normal sexual response. J Sex Med 2009;6:30–9. (Level III)

94. Koski ME, Chermansky CJ. Does estrogen have any real effect on voiding dysfunction in women? Curr Urol Rep 2011;12:345–50. (Level III)

95. Cody JD, Jacobs ML, Richardson K, Moehrer B, Hextall A. Oestrogen therapy for urinary incontinence in post-menopausal women. Cochrane Database of Systematic Revews 2012, Issue 10. Art.No.: CD001405. DOI:10.1002/14651858.CD001405.pub3. (Meta-analysis)

96. Santoro N, Torrens J, Crawford S, Allsworth JE, Finkelstein JS, Gold EB, et al. Correlates of circulating androgens in mid-life women: the study of women's health across the nation. J Clin Endocrinol Metab 2005;90:4836–45. (Level II-3)

97. Davis SR, Davison SL, Donath S, Bell RJ. Circulating androgen levels in self-reported sexual function in women. JAMA 2005;294:91–6. (Level I)

98. Basson R, Brotto LA, Petkau J, Labrie F. Role of androgens in women's sexual dysfunction. Menopause 2010;17:962–71. (Level II-3)

99. Labrie F, Belanger A, Cusan L, Gomez JL, Candas B. Marked decline in serum concentrations of adrenal C19 sex steroid precursors and conjugated

androgen metabolites during aging. J Clin Endocrinol Metab 1997;82:2396–402. (Level III)

100. Davison SL, Bell R, Donath S, Montalto JG, Davis SR. Androgen levels in adult females: changes with age, menopause, and oophorectomy. J Clin Endocrinol Metab 2005;90:3847–53. (Level II-3)

101. Hayes RD. Assessing female sexual dysfunction in epidemiological studies: why is it necessary to measure both low sexual function and sexually related distress? Sex Health 2008;5:215–8. (Level III)

102. Erekson EA, Martin DK, Zhu K, Ciarleglio MM, Patel DA, Guess MK, et al. Sexual function in older women after oophorectomy. Obstet Gynecol 2012;120:833–42. (Level II-3)

103. Melcangi RC, Garcia-Segura LM, Mensah-Nyagan AG. Neuroactive steroids: state of the art and new perspectives. Cell Mol Life Sci 2008;65:777–97. (Level III)

104. Ishunina TA, Swaab DF. Alterations in the human brain in menopause. Maturitas 2007;57:20–2. (Level III)

105. Davis SR, Panjari M, Stanczyk FZ. Clinical review: DHEA replacement for postmenopausal women. J Clin Endocrinol Metab 2011;96:1642–53. (Level III)

106. Genazzani AR, Stomati M, Valentino V, Pluchino N, Pot E, Casarosa E, et al. Effect of 1-year, low-dose DHEA therapy on climacteric symptoms and female sexuality. Climacteric 2011;14:661–8. (Level II-3)

107. Minto CL, Liao KL, Conway GS, Creighton SM. Sexual function in women with complete androgen insensitivity syndrome. Fertil Steril 2003;80:157–64. (Level III)

108. Kohler B, Kleinemeier E, Lux A, Hiort O, Gruters A, Thyen U. Satisfaction with genital surgery and sexual life of adults with XY disorders of sex development: results from the German clinical evaluation study. DDS Network Working Group. J Clin Endocrinol Metab 2012;97: 577–88. (Level III)

109. Braunstein G, Sundwall DA, Katz M, Shifren JL, Buster JE, Simon JA, et al. Safety and efficacy of a testosterone patch for the treatment of hypoactive sexual disorder in surgically menopausal women: a randomized, placebo-controlled trial. Arch Intern Med 2005;165:1582–9. (Level I)

110. Buster JE, Kingsberg SA, Aguirre O, Brown C, Breaux JG, Buch A, et al. Testosterone patch for low sexual desire in surgically menopausal women: a randomized trial. Obstet Gynecol 2005;105:944–52. (Level I)

111. Simon J, Braunstein G, Nachtigall L, Utian W, Katz M, Miller S, et al. Testosterone patch increases sexual activity and desire in surgically menopausal women with hypoactive sexual desire disorder. J Clin Endocrinol Metab 2005;90:5226–33. (Level I)

112. Davis SR, van der Mooren MJ, van Lunsen RH, Lopes P, Ribot C, Rees M, et al. Efficacy and safety of a testosterone patch for the treatment of hypoactive sexual desire disorder in surgically menopausal women: a random-

ized, placebo controlled-trial [published erratum appears in Menopause 2006;13:850]. Menopause 2006;13:387–96. (Level I)

113. White WB, Grady D, Giudice LC, Berry SM, Zborowski J, Snabes MC. A cardiovascular safety study of LibiGel (testosterone gel) in postmenopausal women with elevated cardiovascular risk and hypoactive sexual desire disorder. Am Heart J 2012;163:27–32. (Level I)

114. Snabes MC, Zborowski J, Simes S. Libigel™ (testosterone gel) does not differentiate from placebo therapy in the treatment of hypoactive sexual desire in postmenopausal women [abstract]. J Sex Med 2012;9(suppl):171.

115. Shifren JL, Davis SR, Moreau M, Waldbaum A, Bouchard C, DeRogatis L, et al. Testosterone patch for the treatment of hypoactive sexual desire disorder in naturally menopausal women: results from the INTIMATE NM1 Study [published erratum appears in Menopause 2007;14:157]. Menopause 2006;13:770–9. (Level I)

116. Davis S, Moreau M, Kroll R, Bouchard C, Panay N, Gass M, et al. Testosterone for low libido in postmenopausal women not taking estrogen. APHRODITE Study Team. N Eng J Med 2008;359:2005–17. (Level I)

117. Panay N, Al-Azzawi F, Bouchard C, Davis SR, Eden J, Lodhi I, et al. Testosterone treatment of HSDD in naturally menopausal women: the ADORE study. Climacteric 2010;13:121–31. (Level I)

118. Barton DL, Wender DB, Sloan JA, Dalton RJ, Balcueva EP, Atherton PJ, et al. Randomized controlled trial to evaluate transdermal testosterone in female cancer survivors with decreased libido; North Central Cancer Treatment Group protocol N02C3. J Natl Cancer Inst 2007;99:672–9. (Level I)

119. Wild RA. Endogenous androgens and cardiovascular risk. Menopause 2007; 14:609–10. (Level III)

120. Davis S, Papalia MA, Norman RJ, O'Neill S, Redelman M, Williamson M, et al. Safety and efficacy of a testosterone metered-dose transdermal spray for treating decreased sexual satisfaction in premenopausal women: a randomized trial. Ann Intern Med 2008;148:569–77. (Level I)

121. Davis SR, Nijland FA, Weijmar-Schultz W. Tibolone versus transdermal continuous combined estrogen + progestogen in the treatment of female sexual dysfunction in naturally menopausal women: results from the LISA trial [abstract]. Maturitas 2006;54(suppl):S42–3.

122. BioSante Pharmaceuticals announces positive LibiGel phase III safety date from review and decision to conclude the safety study [press release]. Lincolnshire, IL: Business Wire; February 14, 2011. (Level III)

123. Snabes M, White W, Zborowski J, Berry S. Low cardiovascular event rate in post-menopausal women with increased cardiac risk: updated findings from the ongoing blinded libigel™ (testosterone gel) cardiovascular safety study [abstract]. J Sex Med 2011;8(suppl):16.

124. Davis SR, Braunstein GD. Efficacy and safety of testosterone in the management of hypoactive sexual desire disorder in postmenopausal women. J Sex Med 2012;9:1134–48. (Level III)

125. Arlt W. Androgen therapy in women. Eur J Endocrinol 2006;154: 1–11. (Level III)

126. Bitzer J, Kenemans P, Mueck AO. Breast cancer risk in postmenopausal women using testosterone in combination with hormone replacement therapy. FSDeducation Group. Maturitas 2008;59:209–18. (Level III)

127. Brand JS, van der Schouw YT. Testosterone, SHBG and cardiovascular health in postmenopausal women. Int J Impot Res 2010;22:91–104. (Level II-3)

128. Testosterone patches for female sexual dysfunction. Drug Ther Bull 2009; 47:30–4. (Level III)

129. Hubayter Z, Simon JA. Testosterone therapy for sexual dysfunction in postmenopausal women. Climacteric 2008;11:181–91. (Level III)

130. European Medicines Agency. Intrinsa (testosterone): withdrawal of the marketing authorisation in the European Union. Public statement. London: EMA; 2012. Available at: http://www.ema.europa.eu/docs/en_GB/ document_library/Public_statement/2012/06/WC500128837.pdf. Retrieved February 21, 2014. (Level III)

131. Labrie F, Archer D, Bouchard C, Fortier M, Cusan L, Gomez JL, et al. Effect on intravaginal dehydroepiandrosterone (Prasterone) on libido and sexual dysfunction in postmenopausal women. Menopause 2009;16:923–31. (Level I)

132. Labrie F, Martel C, Berube R, Cote I, Labrie C, Cusan L, et al. Intravaginal prasterone (DHEA) provides local action without clinically significant changes in serum concentrations of estrogens or androgens. J Steroid Biochem Mol Biol 2013;138:359–67. (Level I)

133. Raghunandan C, Agrawal S, Dubey P, Choudhury M, Jain A. A comparative study of the effects of local estrogen with or without local testosterone on vulvovaginal and sexual dysfunction in postmenopausal women. J Sex Med 2010;7:1284–90. (Level I)

134. World Health Organization. The ICD-10 classification of mental and behavioural disorders: clinical descriptions and diagnostic guidelines. Geneva: WHO; 1992. Available at: http://www.who.int/classifications/icd/en/bluebook.pdf. Retrieved January 24, 2014. (Level III)

135. Basson R, Schultz WW. Sexual sequelae of general medical disorders. Lancet 2007;369:409–24. (Level III)

136. Khandker M, Brady SS, Vitonis AF, MacLehose RF, Stewart EG, Harlow BL. The influence of depression and anxiety on risk of adult onset vulvodynia. J Women's Health (Larchmt) 2011;20:1445–51. (Level II-3)

137. Basson R. Sexual function of women with chronic illness and cancer. Womens Health (Lond Engl) 2010;6:407–29. (Level III)

138. Nusbaum MR, Gamble G, Skinner B, Heiman J. The high prevalence of sexual concerns among women seeking routine gynecological care. J Fam Pract 2000;49:229–32. (Level II-3)

139. Leonard LM, Follette VM. Sexual functioning in women reporting a history of sexual child abuse: review of the empirical literature and clinical implications. Annu Rev Sex Res 2002;13:346–88. (Level III)

140. Staples J, Rellini AH, Roberts SP. Avoiding experiences: sexual dysfunction in women with a history of sexual abuse in childhood and adolescence. Arch Sex Behav 2012;41:341–50. (Level II-2)

141. Bitzer J, Brandenburg U. Psychotherapeutic interventions for female sexual dysfunction. Maturitas 2009;63:160–3. (Level III)

142. Bradford A, Meston CM. Behavior and symptom change among women treated with placebo for sexual dysfunction. J Sex Med 2011;8:191–201. (Level II-3)

143. Brotto LA, Basson R, Luria M. A mindfulness-based group psychoeducational intervention targeting sexual arousal disorder in women. J Sex Med 2008;5:1646–59. (Level III)

144. Brotto L, Heiman J, Goff B, Greer B, Lentz GM, Swisher E, et al. A psychoeducational intervention for sexual dysfunction in women with gynecologic cancer. Arch Sex Behav 2008; 37:317–29. (Level II-3)

145. Brotto L. Mindfulness applications to women's sexual dysfunction: applications for low desire, sexual distress, and provoked vestibulodynia [abstract]. J Sex Med 2011;8(suppl 3):94. (Level III)

146. Brotto LA, Basson R, Carlson M, Zhu C. Impact of an integrated mindfulness and cognitive behavioural treatment for provoked vestibulodynia (IMPROVED): a qualitative study. Sex Relation Ther 2013;28:3–19. (Level III)

147. Zeidan F, Martucci KT, Kraft RA, McHaffie JG, Coghill RC. Neural correlates of mindfulness meditation-related anxiety relief. Soc Cogn Affect Neurosci 2013. DOI: 10.1093/sca/nst041. (Level III)

148. Zeidan F, Martucci KT, Kraft RA, Gordon NS, McHaffie JG, Coghill RC. Brain mechanisms supporting the modulation of pain by mindfulness meditation. J Neurosci 2011;31:5540–8. (Level III)

149. Ives-Deliperi VL, Solms M, Meintjes EM. The neural substrates of mindfulness: an fMRI investigation. Soc Neurosci 2011;6:231–42. (Level III)

150. Middleton LS, Kuffel SW, Heiman JR. Effects of experimentally adopted sexual schemas on vaginal response and subjective sexual arousal: a comparison between women with arousal disorder and sexually healthy women. Arch Sex Behav 2008;37:950–61. (Level II-3)

151. Nobre PJ. Determinants of sexual desire problems in women: testing a cognitive-emotional model. J Sex Marit Ther 2009;35:360–77. (Level II-3)

152. Brotto LA, Petkau AJ, Labrie F, Basson R. Predictors of sexual desire disorders in women. J Sex Med 2011;8;742–53. (Level II-3)

153. Basson R, Smith KB. Incorporating mindfulness meditation into the treatment of povoked vestibulodynia. Curr Sex Health Rep 2014;6:20–9.

154. Fruhauf S, Gerger H, Schmidt HM, Munder T, Barth J. Efficacy of psychological interventions for sexual dysfunction: a systematic review and meta-analysis. Arch Sex Behav 2013;42:915–33. (Meta-analysis)

155. Taylor S, Harley C, Ziegler L, Brown J, Velikova G. Interventions for sexual problems following treatment for breast cancer: a systematic review. Breast Cancer Res Treat 2011;130:711–24. (Level II-3)

156. Wierman ME, Nappi RE, Avis N, Davis SR, Labrie F, Rosner W, et al. Endocrine aspects of women's sexual function J Sex Med 2010;7:561–85. (Level III)

157. Nurnberg HG, Hensley PL, Heiman JR, Croft HA, Debattista C, Paine S. Sildenafil treatment of women with antidepressant-associated sexual dysfunction: a randomized controlled trial. JAMA 2008;300:395–404. (Level I)

158. Schroder M, Mell LK, Hurteau JA, Collins YC, Rotmensch J, Waggoner SE, et al. Clitoral therapy device for treatment of sexual dysfunction in irradiated cervical cancer patients. Int J Radiat Oncol Biol Phys 2005;61:1078–86. (Level III)

159. Heiman JR. Orgasmic disorders in women. In: Leiblum SR, editor. Principles and practice of sex therapy. 4th ed. New York (NY): Guilford Press; 2007. p. 84–123. (Level III)

160. Trudel G, Marchand A, Ravart M, Aubin S, Turgeon L, Fortier P. The effect of a cognitive-behavioral group treatment program on hypoactive sexual desire in women. Sex Rel Ther 2001;16:145–64. (Level II-3)

161. Killmann PR, Mills KH, Caid C, Davidson E, Bella B, Milan R, et al. Treatment of secondary orgasmic dysfunction: an outcome study. Arch Sex Behav 1986;15:211–29. (Level III)

162. Spence SH. Group versus individual treatment of primary and secondary female orgasmic dysfunction. Behav Res Ther 1985;23:539–48. (Level I)

163. Meston CM, Hull E, Levin RJ, Sipski M. Disorders of orgasm in women. J Sex Med 2004;1:66–8. (Level III)

164. Hurlbert DF, Apt C. The coital alignment technique and directed masturbation: a comparative study on female orgasm. J Sex Marital Ther 1995;21: 21–9. (Level I)

165. Simon JA. Identifying and treating sexual dysfunction in postmenopausal women: the role of estrogen. J Womens Health (Larchmt) 2011;20:1453–65. (Level III)

166. Chen J, Geng L, Song X, Li H, Giordan N, Liao Q. Evaluation of the efficacy and safety of hyaluronic acid vaginal gel to ease vaginal dryness: a multicenter, randomized, controlled, open-label, parallel-group, clinical trial. J Sex Med 2013;10:1575–84. (Level I)

167. Huang AJ, Moore EE, Boyko EJ, Scholes D, Lin F, Vittinghoff E, et al. Vaginal symptoms in post menopausal women: self-reported severity, natural history, and risk factors. Menopause 2010;17:121–6. (Level II-3)

168. Indhavivadhana S, Leerasiri P, Rattanachaiyanont M, Laiwejpithaya S, Tanmahasamut P, Techatraisak K, et al. Vaginal atrophy and sexual

dysfunction in current users of systemic postmenopausal hormone therapy. J Med Assoc Thai 2010;93:667–75. (Level III)

169. Kao A, Binik YM, Amsel R, Funaro D, Leroux N, Khalife S. Challenging atrophied perspectives on postmenopausal dyspareunia: a systematic description and synthesis of clinical pain characteristics. J Sex Marital Ther 2012;38:128–50. (Level II-3)

170. Rossouw JE, Anderson GL, Prentice RL, LaCroix AZ, Kooperberg C, Stefanick ML, et al. Risks and benefits of estrogen plus progestin in healthy women: principal results from the Women's Health Initiative randomized controlled trial. Writing Group for the Women's Health Initiative Investigators. JAMA 2002;288:321–33. (Level I)

171. Desrochers G, Bergeron S, Landry T, Jodoin M. Do psychosexual factors play a role in the etiology of provoked vestibulodynia? A critical review. J Sex Marital Ther 2008;34:198–226. (Level III)

172. Tracey I, Bushnell MC. How neuroimaging studies have challenged us to rethink: is chronic pain a disease? J Pain 2009;10:1113–20. (Level III)

173. Schweinhardt P, Kuchinad A, Pukall CF, Bushnell MC. Increase gray matter density in young women with chronic vulvar pain. Pain 2008;140:411–9. (Level II-3)

174. Gunter J. Vulvodynia: new thoughts on a devastating condition. Obstet Gynecol Surv 2007;62:812–8. (Level III)

175. Foster DC, Kotok MB, Huang LS, Watts A, Oakes D, Howard FM, et al. Oral desipramine and topical lidocaine for vulvodynia: a randomized controlled trial. Obstet Gynecol 2010;116:583–93. (Level I)

176. Leo RJ. A systematic review of the utility of anticonvulsant pharmacotherapy in the treatment of vulvodynia pain. J Sex Med 2013;10:2000–8. (Level III)

177. Tommola P, Unkila-Kallio L, Paavonen J. Surgical treatment of vulvar vestibulitis: a review. Acta Obstet Gynecol Scand 2010;89:1385–95. (Level III)

178. Heddini U, Bohm-Starke N, Nilsson KW, Johannesson U. Provoked vestibulodynia--medical factors and comorbidity associated with treatment outcome. J Sex Med 2012;9:1400–6. (Level III)

179. Gwilym SE, Keltner JR, Warnaby CE, Carr AJ, Chizh B, Chessell I, et al. Psychophysical and functional imaging evidence supporting the presence of central sensitization in a cohort of osteoarthritis patients. Arthritis Rheum 2009;61:1226–34. (Level II-3)

180. Hampson JP, Reed BD, Clauw DJ, Bhavsar R, Gracely RH, Haefner HK, et al. Augmented central pain processing in vulvodynia. J Pain 2013;14:579–89. (Level II-3)

181. Giesecke J, Reed BD, Haefner KH, Giesecke T, Clauw DJ, Gracely RH. Quantitative sensory testing in vulvodynia patients and increased peripheral pressure pain sensitivity. Obstet Gynecol 2004;104:126–33. (Level II-3)

182. Brown CA, Jones AK. Meditation experience predicts less negative appraisal of pain: electrophysiological evidence for the involvement of anticipatory neural responses. Pain 2010;150:428–38. (Level III)

183. Grant JA, Courtemanche J, Rainville P. A non-elaborative mental stance and decoupling of executive and pain-related cortices predicts low pain sensitivity in Zen meditators. Pain 2011;152:150–6. (Level III)

184. Chiesa A, Brambilla P, Serretti A. Functional neural correlates of mindfulness meditations in comparison with psychotherapy, pharmacotherapy and placebo effects. Is there a link? Acta Neuropsychiatr 2010;22:104–17. (Level III)

185. Miner M, Eposito KE, Guay A, Montorsi P, Goldstein I. Cardiometabolic risk and female sexual health: the Princeton III summary. J Sex Med 2012;9:641–51; quiz 652. (Level III)

186. Majerovitz SD, Revenson TA. Sexuality and rheumatic disease: the significance of gender. Arthritis Care Res 1994;7:29–34. (Level III)

187. Abdel-Nasser AM, Ali EI. Determinants of sexual disability and dissatisfaction in female patients with rheumatoid arthritis. Clin Rheumatol 2006;25:822–30. (Level II-3)

188. Hibbard MR, Gordon WA, Flanagan S, Haddad L, Labinsky E. Sexual dysfunction after traumatic brain injury. Neurorehabilitation 2000;15:107–20. (Level II-3)

189. Meco G, Rubino A, Caravona N, Valente M. Sexual dysfunction in Parkinson's disease. Parkinsonism Relat Disord 2008;14:451–6. (Level III)

190. Hulter BM, Lundberg PO. Sexual function in women with advanced multiple sclerosis. J Neurol Neurosurg Psychiatry 1995;59:83–6. (Level III)

191. Komisaruk BR, Whipple B, Crawford A, Liu WC, Kalnin A, Mosier K. Brain activation during vaginocervical self-stimulation and orgasm in women with complete spinal cord injury: fMRI evidence of mediation by the vagus nerves. Brain Res 2004;1024:77–88. (Level III)

192. Ekland MB, Krassioukov AV, McBride KE, Eliott SL. Incidence of autonomic dysreflexia and silent autonomic dysreflexia in men with spinal cord injury undergoing sperm retrieval: implications for clinical practice. J Spinal Cord Med 2008;31:33–9. (Level III)

193. Bhasin S, Enzlin P, Caviello A, Basson R. Sexual dysfunction in men and women with endocrine disorders. Lancet 2007;369:597–611. (Level III)

194. Ponholzer A, Temml C, Rauchenwald M, Marszalek M, Madersbacher S. Is the metabolic syndrome a risk factor for female sexual dysfunction in sexually active women? Int J Impot Res 2008;20:100–4. (Level II-3)

195. Servoss SJ, Januzzi JL, Muller JE. Triggers of acute coronary syndromes. Prog Cardiovasc Dis 2002;44:369–42. (Level III)

196. Krychman ML, Katz A. Breast cancer and sexuality: multi-modal treatment options. J Sex Med 2012;9:5–13; quiz 14–5. (Level III)

197. Baumgart J, Nilsson K, Evers AS, kallak TK, Poromaa IS. Sexual dysfunction in women with adjuvant endocrine therapy after breast cancer. Menopause 2013;20:162–8. (Level III)

198. Kendall A, Dowsett M, Folkerd E, Smith I. Caution: vaginal estradiol appears to be contraindicated in postmenopausal women on adjunct aromatase inhibitors. Ann Oncol 2006;17:584–7. (Level III)

199. Boehmer U, Timm A, Ozonoff A, Potter J. Explanatory factors of sexual function in sexual minority women breast cancer survivors. Ann Oncol 2012;23:2873–8. (Level II-3)

200. Gilbert E, Ussher JM, Perz J. Sexuality after gynaecological cancer: a review of the material, intrapsychic, and discursive aspects of treatment on women's sexual-wellbeing. Maturitas 2011;70:42–57. (Level III)

201. Jensen PT, Groenvold M, Klee MC, Thranov I, Petersen MA, Machin D. Early stage cervical carcinoma, radical hysterectomy and sexual functioning. Cancer 2004;100:97–106. (Level II-3)

202. Abbott-Anderson K, Kwekkeboom KL. A syematic review of sexual concerns reported by gynecological cancer survivors [published erratum appears in Gynecol Oncol 2012;126:501–8]. Gynecol Oncol 2012;124:477–89. (Level III)

203. Cullen K, Fergus K, Dasgupta D, Fitch M, Doyle C, Adams L. From "sex toy" to intrusive imposition: a qualitative examination of women's experiences with daily dilator use following treatment for gynecological cancer. J Sex Med 2012;9:1162–73. (Level III)

204. Brotto LA, Erskine Y, Carey M, Ehlen T, Finlayson S, Heywood M, et al. A brief mindfulness-based cognitive behavioral intervention improves sexual functioning versus wait-list control in women treated for gynecologic cancer. Gynecol Oncol 2012;125:320–5. (Level III)

205. Maughan K, Clarke C. The effect of a clinical nurse specialist in gynaecological oncology on quality of life and sexuality. J Clin Nurs 2001;10:221–9. (Level I)

206. Ito TY, Polan ML, Whipple B, Trant AS. The enhancement of female sexual function with ArginMax, a nutritional supplement, among women differing in menopausal status. J Sex Marit Ther 2006;32:369–78. (Level I)

207. Leddy LS, Yang CC, Stuckey BG, Sudworth M, Haughie S, Sultana S, et al. Influence of sildenafil on genital engorgement in women with female sexual arousal disorder. J Sex Med 2012;9:2693–7. (Level I)

208. Ferguson DM, Hosmane B, Heiman JR. Randomized, placebo-controlled, double-blind, parallel design trial of the efficacy and safety of Zestra in women with mixed sexual desire/interest/arousal/orgasm disorders. J Sex Marit Ther 2010;36:66–86. (Level I)

209. Soe LH, Wurz GT, Kao CJ, DeGregorio MW. Ospemifene for the treatment of dyspareunia associated with vulvar and vaginal atrophy: potential benefits in bone and breast. Int J Womens Health 2013;5:605–11. (Level III)

210. Mirkin S, Komm BS. Tissue-selective estrogen complexes for postmenopausal women. Maturitas 2013;76:213–20. (Level III)

Studies were reviewed and evaluated for quality according to the method outlined by the U.S. Preventive Services Task Force:

I　　Evidence obtained from at least one properly designed randomized controlled trial.

II-1　Evidence obtained from well-designed controlled trials without randomization.

II-2　Evidence obtained from well-designed cohort or case–control analytic studies, preferably from more than one center or research group.

II-3　Evidence obtained from multiple time series with or without the intervention. Dramatic results in uncontrolled experiments also could be regarded as this type of evidence.

III　　Opinions of respected authorities, based on clinical experience, descriptive studies, or reports of expert committees.

Answers

1. C, 2. B, 3. A, 4. B, 5. D, 6. B, 7. D, 8. B, 9. B, 10. C, 11. B, 12. B, 13. A, 14. C

Index

Forthcoming Titles

Each monograph in *Clinical Updates in Women's Health Care* is an overview of a topic of importance to obstetrician–gynecologists in practice. Upcoming titles include the following:

- Nutrition
- Adverse Drug Reactions
- Memory Loss and Dementia
- Office Emergencies
- Metabolic Bone Disease
- Benign Breast Disease
- Lower Gastrointestinal Tract Disorders

If not previously completed, earn CME credits for back issues of *Clinical Updates in Women's Health Care*. Listed are recent titles. For a complete list of titles, visit www.clinicalupdates.org.

- *Obesity* (Volume XII, Number 1, January 2013)
- *Exercise* (Volume XII, Number 2, April 2013)
- *Diabetes Mellitus* (Volume XII, Number 3, July 2013)
- *Allergies* (Volume XII, Number 4, October 2013)
- *Thyroid Disorders* (Volume XII, Number 5, November 2013)
- *Autoimmune Disorders* (Volume XIII, Number 1, January 2014)

You can sign up for a 1-year subscription to *Clinical Updates in Women's Health Care* at the rate of $65 for College members ($115 nonmembers). Individual copies also can be purchased for $25 ($35 nonmembers). You can subscribe by calling (800) 762-2264 or online at sales.acog.org. Online access is available to subscribers at www.clinicalupdates.org.

The Editorial Board welcomes comments and suggestions for topics. Please contact the Editorial Board in care of College Publications (publication@acog.org).

Test Your Clinical Skills—and Earn CME Credits

ACCME Accreditation

The American College of Obstetricians and Gynecologists is accredited by the Accreditation Council for Continuing Medical Education (ACCME) to provide continuing medical education for physicians.

AMA PRA Category 1 Credit(s)™

The American College of Obstetricians and Gynecologists designates this enduring activity for a maximum of 5 AMA PRA Category 1 Credit(s)™. Physicians should only claim credit commensurate with the extent of their participation in the activity.

College Cognate Credit(s)

The American College of Obstetricians and Gynecologists designates this enduring activity for a maximum of 5 Category 1 College Cognate Credit(s). The College has a reciprocity agreement with the AMA that allows *AMA PRA Category 1 Credit(s)*™ to be equivalent to College Cognate Credits.

Credit for *Clinical Updates in Women's Health Care: Sexuality and Sexual Disorders*, Volume XIII, Number 2, April 2014, is initially available through December 2017. During that year, the unit will be reevaluated. If the content remains current, credit is extended for an additional 3 years.

Actual time spent completing this activity (you may record up to 5 hours):_____.

To obtain credits, complete and return this answer sheet to the address shown below (only original answer sheets will be accepted for credit) or submit your answers online at www.clinicalupdates.org:

1. _____   6. _____   11. _____
2. _____   7. _____   12. _____
3. _____   8. _____   13. _____
4. _____   9. _____   14. _____
5. _____   10. _____

ACOG ID Number _ _ _ _ _ _ _ _ _ _ _ _

Name _____

Address_____

City/State/Zip _____

The American College of Obstetricians and Gynecologists
Educational Development and Testing
409 12th Street, SW
PO Box 96920, Washington, DC 20090-6920

Reliable Take-Home Information for Your Patients

The American College of Obstetricians and Gynecologists' Patient Education Pamphlets are designed to complement and supplement the information and advice you provide in the office. After you talk to your patients about sexuality and sexual disorders, ensure they have accurate information they can refer to and share with their families and friends when they are at home.

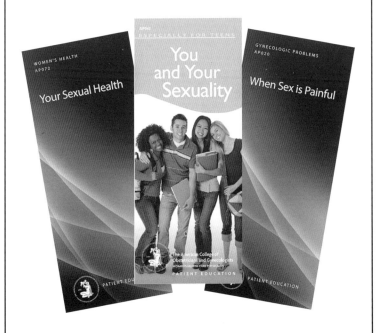